Chronic Fatigue Syndrome

YOUR ROUTE TO RECOVERY

For you, Dad (1966–2021)

Chronic Fatigue Syndrome

YOUR ROUTE TO RECOVERY

Solutions to Lift the Fog
and Light the Way

Lauren Windas

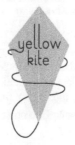

yellow
kite

First published in Great Britain in 2023 by Yellow Kite
An imprint of Hodder & Stoughton
An Hachette UK company

4

Copyright © Lauren Windas 2023

Illustrations on pp. 54, 175 and 281 from shutterstock.com;
on pp. 41, 86, 92, 105, 107, 110, 222, 225, 226
and 260 by Goldust Design; on pp. 43, 46, 47, 48,
85, 99, 170, 265, 267 and 275 by Nicole Windas

A CIP catalogue record for this title is available
from the British Library

Trade Paperback ISBN 978 1 529 37655 5
eBook ISBN 978 1 529 37657 9

Typeset in Magneta by Goldust Design

Printed and bound in Great Britain by Clays Ltd, Elcograf S.p.A.

Hodder & Stoughton policy is to use papers that are
natural, renewable and recyclable products and made from
wood grown in sustainable forests. The logging and manufacturing
processes are expected to conform to the environmental
regulations of the country of origin.

Yellow Kite
Hodder & Stoughton Ltd
Carmelite House
50 Victoria Embankment
London EC4Y 0DZ
www.yellowkitebooks.co.uk

CONTENTS

The terms CFS (chronic fatigue syndrome) and ME (myalgic enceph-alomyelitis) are often used interchangeably, although some professionals do consider them to be slightly different conditions. For the purposes of this book and the avoidance of confusion, however, I will refer to CFS throughout.

While this book is intended to provide a framework of suggestions and strategies for you to explore, it is recommended that you consult with your doctor about any health concern which may require diagnosis and before implementing any of the suggested dietary or lifestyle changes. It may also be worthwhile seeking the one-to-one support of a nutritional therapist, naturopath, and someone who is psychologically-trained such as a psychologist, NLP practitioner, cognitive behavioural ther-apist or hypnotherapist who can support you, alongside your doctor.

Any new symptoms that arise along your recovery journey should also be discussed with your doctor. If you have a history of an eating disorder, do not attempt to remove foods from your diet and please seek professional one-to-one support regarding your nutrition.

The author and publisher disclaim any liability directly or indirectly from the use of the material in this book by any person.

INTRODUCTION

Writing a book about one of the most complex and misunderstood chronic illnesses of modern times feels like an enormous responsibility, but having become unwell with chronic fatigue syndrome (CFS) in 2012, and having since made huge strides in my recovery, I am now passionate about compiling my experiences and research into one place, so that I can pass on my learnings to those caught at the epicentre of this life-altering illness.

This is the book that I wish I'd had at my fingertips all those years ago, before I knew what I do now. Packed with useful information and practical tools, it will be your guide on your recovery journey, saving you hours of endless research at a time when energy is so scarce.

For those of you who are going through this illness, I stand with you. Each and every single one of you is a warrior. And to those close family members or friends affected indirectly by this horrific condition, you are also fighters and your support for your loved one is indispensable.

You may be wondering about the 'fog' of the subtitle: this came to me during a meditation experience. For me, it encapsulates all that CFS is: a murky haze of fog, both in terms of its symptoms and its stigma. The fog is a world in which the condition itself is often overlooked and misunderstood by society and modern medicine alike, so I wanted to write a book that would validate it, acknowledging it for what it truly is, as well as its impact on those who are affected by it. Additionally, one of my worst symptoms was brain fog, and I am eternally grateful that my mind is now in a much clearer place, allowing me to be able to piece all the information together and write this book for you.

So what is CFS?

Chronic fatigue syndrome (CFS)/myalgic encephalomyelitis (ME) is an illness that affects the nervous, immune, digestive and many other body systems, resulting in chronic exhaustion and numerous other debilitating symptoms.

I have read a description of CFS as being 'total or near-total physical and psychological body-breakdown syndrome', where the body is unable to recover following a medical trigger, such as a virus, leaving the sufferer in a perpetual state of ill health. Alongside the severe and persistent fatigue, common features include a whole range of symptoms from cognitive impairment and heart palpitations to painful muscles/joints and gastrointestinal issues, with many others in between (see p. 28 for a more comprehensive list).

The illness is also blighted by both social stigma and a lack of professional understanding, making it even harder to deal with. I know this all too well. My friends never understood and neither did the doctors. Which makes it an incredibly hard place to be, when you are lost within the world of health and medicine, not knowing where to turn for answers or support. And to compound things, no two sufferers deal with the exact same set of symptoms – people can experience CFS to different degrees and symptoms can fluctuate on a daily basis.

About this book

Let's first take a look at what this book *is*:

- A practical, evidence-based guide to accompany those on their own journeys towards recovery from CFS, featuring my personal story, anecdotes, experience of working with clients and contextualisation of research, medical theories and understanding around the condition.

- A toolkit for those who are at a loss as to where to start finding answers, complete with references to publications and studies.

- A source of hope and a guiding light – a hand for you to hold, your best friend to walk with you, each and every step of the way.

- A resource for answers. Because when you are going through CFS, answers are what you want – confirmation that you are not going crazy and that there really is something going on physically to explain your multiple chronic symptoms.

And now, what it *isn't*:

- A cure-all. Each of us is unique and our journeys will not all follow the same path.

The book is divided into three parts.

- In Part 1, I relate my personal experience of CFS, following an infection at university; I describe the path I followed and the changes I made to my lifestyle to recover my health.

- In Part 2, we look at the science: we cover what CFS actually is in more detail – the causes and symptoms, who it affects and how it is diagnosed and treated, among other things.

- Part 3 paves your road to recovery. I outline the model of Functional Medicine (FM, a system of integrative healthcare that examines how and why chronic illness occurs, assessing the root causes of CFS) and provide practical tips, lifestyle advice and techniques for you to reclaim your health and get yourself back on track.

Through my own experiences and studies, I have acquired a thorough understanding of the human body (both on a personal and professional level) – about what it means to be ill and to be well – and now I want to share this wealth of knowledge with you, to make you feel better in your own skin and recover from chronic fatigue.

With this book as your guide, I want you to approach your health like a jigsaw puzzle, finding all the necessary pieces to put together in your recovery. It may be a process of trial and error as you uncover the blocks to your healing, but we will get there together as you take each step forward.

Ultimately, as you learn more about your own unique body and its requirements and take responsibility for your health, I will show you that amid the struggle there is always hope.

Time for a pause ⏸

As you work your way through the book, you will intermittently come across this 'pause' symbol: ⏸. I am aware that many of you in the CFS community might find it challenging at times to digest certain sections (particularly those of you who experience brain fog), so these 'pauses' are conveniently placed to allow you to take stock, rest, breathe and then come back to the information that is relevant to you, to help you better understand your condition. Use these to your advantage, as you work your way through the book, so that you are in the best possible place to benefit from it.

PART 1
My Story

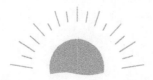

This first part of the book is about my personal experience of battling CFS, and the path I embarked on to reclaim my health.

Despite my health struggles, it was a journey of self-discovery, as I came to understand more about this complex chronic illness that can profoundly change the lives of those who suffer with it. It sparked a passion to share my learnings with others, and I hope that I can be a voice of trust and understanding, given that I have walked in your shoes.

Let's begin . . .

CHAPTER 1

A Personal Journey

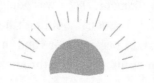

Life is a balance between holding on and letting go.
Rumi, thirteenth-century Persian poet

There is something particularly vulnerable about opening up to people you don't know and laying yourself bare, but, in order to express the nature of what I do, I must first tell you my story.

It was September 2012, and I was beginning my second year at university at the tender age of nineteen. I couldn't wait to return to student life.

I loved the atmosphere in Newcastle; it definitely gets my vote as the best student city! Everywhere you turned there was something going on: bar crawls, socials, student nights, you name it – Newcastle is most definitely set up for the young and lively.

My first year of university had been one of the best of my life. I wasn't the most confident girl in the world, but I think I must have been struck by luck in terms of who I was with in my halls and on my English Literature course; forming connections with those around me seemed so effortless, as I met the most incredible people and made some amazing memories, cementing my first years of adulthood and independence. Not only did I make wonderful new friends, I was also lucky in that my best friends from school joined me there, too. And what's more, my older sister, Nicole, was there as well.

So as you can imagine, my first year having gone down without a hitch, as I embarked on the second I was elated to be moving out of student halls and into a flat with two friends and my sister. I felt even more grown up and independent than ever.

It was the first week back after the summer holidays, and I was not feeling quite right. It was a very strange and surreal time for me. I was sitting in the living room with my friends and something hit me like a wave – dread. I had never experienced it before, but I knew I was having a panic attack. The only way I can describe the feeling is that I thought, in that very moment, that I was going to die. I have no idea why, as it was completely irrational, but that's how I felt. As the sensation rose within me, and I became more and more anxious, I quickly darted out of the room, went into the bathroom and tried to take some deep breaths.

Having waited it out in the bathroom, I tried to carry on with my day, but a sense of unease was still there. I couldn't stop thinking about it. It was as though something within me had broken and I didn't know what it was or why it had happened.

A few days later I was hit by another blow, when my boyfriend nearly broke up with me. As you can imagine, 'first-love syndrome' got the better of me. I was absolutely devastated at the possibility of losing him, and it's safe to say that the stress of it all contributed to me catching a viral infection that just wouldn't shift.

Over the next few weeks, I would regularly throw my head over bowls of steaming hot water and bathe myself in VapoRub, trying to clear what felt like the most intense flu I had ever experienced. As the weeks passed, I just couldn't believe that I still wasn't getting any better. If anything, my symptoms had started to get worse. I was struggling to climb out of bed in the mornings. I would wake up tired, with severe muscle pain and soreness, as though I had run a marathon the day before, and I felt dizzy and light-headed every time I tried to stand up.

At this point I felt that some intervention was necessary, so I went along to the doctor for some help. Despite the consensus of a viral infection, I was treated with a two-week course of antibiotics and advised to go back to my home in East Yorkshire and rest.

So back home I went. I spent my days relishing my mum's care and enjoying not having to worry about cooking, cleaning or studying.

Instead, I spent endless hours devouring TV programmes and focused on getting myself better, so that I could return to my exciting life at uni.

Three weeks passed and the main symptoms of flu I'd been experiencing, such as a cough and stuffy nose, seemed to disappear. Great news, I thought, and off I went back to Newcastle. However, I was disheartened to still feel under the weather upon my return. I was showing up to lectures half-asleep, feeling as though I just wanted to curl up into a ball and snooze. I would sit in the lecture auditorium, clock-watching, waiting for my next free period so I could go back to my room and collapse under the duvet.

Friends would check in on me to see if I was feeling any better. 'There's definitely something going around,' they'd say. Or, 'It's probably just taking a little while to clear, that's all. You'll be right as rain soon enough.' Initially, I thought they were right – that it was probably just one of those nasty viruses that takes hold for four to six weeks. But as the weeks went on, I wasn't so sure. I couldn't put my finger on what was wrong. I just didn't feel 'present', for want of a better word. I didn't feel real. It was as though there was a haze or a fog preventing me from being able to think clearly. And wherever I looked, it was there.

Everything I did demanded that much more effort to process. And the heavy reading load of an English Literature degree certainly didn't help. For each module, I was tasked with reading chapters of various books, from James Joyce's 730-page *Ulysses* to Robert Louis Stevenson's *The Strange Case of Dr Jekyll and Mr Hyde*. It was tricky at the best of times, as I am *not* the quickest reader. But with a foggy brain, I might as well have given up.

I also remember going completely blank in the middle of conversations with friends. It was like having the brain of a seventy-year-old in a nineteen-year-old's body. It was mortifying and terrifying all at the same time.

Other strange symptoms soon reared their heads, such as feeling completely exhausted after any physical or mental activity. Initially, I thought it was just physical exertion that caused the fatigue. But soon I realised that I had an incredibly low stress threshold. So at the first sign of any pressure – say, from an upcoming uni deadline – I would be in a fit of panic, experiencing heart palpitations, sweating and crying spells, which left me feeling completely depleted.

On top of all this, my digestive system was an absolute mess. I had suffered with IBS since the age of fourteen, yet the toilet topic was a *huge* taboo for me, and I avoided discussing it at all costs. I had always felt embarrassed about my symptoms, never uttering a word about them to my friends. But now the IBS became more debilitating than ever, and it just seemed that my health was on a downward spiral. It was all so scary, and my mood was starting to take a big hit, too.

I had never thought of myself as a 'sick' person before. You know, the ones who are always absent from events, struck down by something or other. Until then, I had always been relatively healthy. In fact, in my social circle, I would have considered myself the healthiest. I was active and would normally visit the gym three to four times a week. I followed a pescatarian diet. I had never been through anything like this before.

So back to the doctor I went. I couldn't help but wonder what the GP was going to do to help me, but as I sat in the cold, uncomfortable waiting room – a place that tends to make most people feel sick and anxious – I nevertheless felt pure hope and optimism. A doctor's job is to get you better, after all, I thought.

My name flashed up on the digital screen, and I walked into the GP's room and told her how I was feeling. She had me tested for everything under the sun. Lyme disease – negative; glandular fever – negative; coeliac disease – negative . . . The list went on, with no answers as to what was happening to me, leaving me feeling incredibly lost and very alone.

I ended up hopping from one GP to the next, for second and third opinions, listing my various symptoms, including fatigue, brain fog, muscle pains, gas, bloating and nausea, diarrhoea, temperature sensitivities, dizziness, vertigo and heart palpitations.

I saw countless GPs and specialists, but not one was able to say what was wrong with me. Meanwhile, I tried to continue as a typical student, but I felt largely disassociated and concerns about my health were making student life increasingly strained.

I eventually made a trip down to Harley Street in London, where a consultant mentioned the words chronic fatigue syndrome to me, although no formal diagnosis was made.

After that appointment, I went online and searched chronic fatigue syndrome, but I had to close the internet browser because it induced utter terror, fear and devastation. Yes, I was able to marry my symptoms up as an exact match with what I found there – but seeing the words 'no cure' and the fact that I might have to live with this illness for the rest of my life was a prospect I refused to accept.

The start of the journey

As 2013 dawned, my amazing mother shone a light on an alternative approach.

To tell you a little bit about my mum, she is the most caring woman you could ever meet. Following endless hours of extensive research and trawling the internet, she introduced me to the field of nutrition and naturopathy, where I began my quest to reclaim my health.

At the time, I had zero understanding of what naturopathy was, and the alternative-medicine approach all sounded a bit weird and wacky to me. I quickly learned, however, that naturopathy is a mode of lifestyle medicine that promotes wellbeing by addressing the root cause of a health problem. It considers the triggers of poor health and how people can make lifestyle changes to prompt the body's self-healing mechanisms to return it to its natural state of optimum health.

So the mode for dealing with my chronic illness was to be, it seemed, through lifestyle medicine. And despite my qualms, I had no option but to take this route because conventional medicine was offering me nothing, and I was terrified of feeling this way for ever.

Determined to get well again, I spent time consulting with a naturopath to put the puzzle pieces together of what was causing my ill health. In our first consultation, we spent most of the time talking about my digestive system: how many bowel movements I had each day, what the form was like – even the smell. Me being me, I couldn't help but giggle through my embarrassment over answering his various questions.

Most of the consultation was geared towards my gut, and I kept thinking, But I am tired all the time and my brain is foggy! However, he soon went on to bridge the apparent gap, explaining that my digestive system was involved in various other symptoms, and that he therefore wanted to examine the ecology of my gut through a stool test to detect any underlying imbalances.

I understood that I had digestive issues, but I saw these as separate from my symptoms of fatigue and brain fog, remaining convinced that a virus had been the straw that broke the camel's back. Yet I remembered a television interview with actress Cameron Diaz, who talked very openly about how our poo can say a lot about our overall health, and I could see this was fast becoming a topic of conversation.

So there I was, facing the discomfort of pooing into a sample pot and posting it back to the lab – I was clearly going to do whatever it took! The test wasn't cheap either, but I was very fortunate in that my parents could afford to support me in paying for it. I was praying for any answers that it could give me, providing a straightforward resolution to my problem.

The results came back and showed that I had some imbalances in the communities of microorganisms living inside me – something known as 'dysbiosis'. My stool test result showed high levels of pathogenic bacteria and Candida albicans – a type of yeast that can overgrow and create havoc in the gut, leading to symptoms such as fatigue and digestive issues. On top of this, the report also indicated the presence of two parasites that thrive off sugar, and – much to my dismay – I was told to embark on a strict sugar-free diet as a mode of addressing this. I was also advised to take some natural anti-microbial supplements, which would work to combat the imbalances within my gut.

Now, I have always loved food. It is something that undeniably brings people together and, like everybody else, I would often celebrate life with food. So being told that my health problems needed to be tackled through diet was one of the most daunting things for me to hear.

Nevertheless, I was elated to know that I wasn't going crazy and that there was indeed something wrong with me.

Gut feeling

I came to discover that the state of my gut was at the root of a lot of the chronic symptoms I was experiencing, and that dysbiosis, antibiotic use, parasites, stress, the oral contraceptive pill and a poor diet all played a part.

It's funny because, while IBS had been with me since the age of fourteen, and the telltale signs were there all along, it was only the debilitating chronic fatigue and brain fog that made me start to look in the right direction and, ultimately, address my gut health. In the first few months of becoming unwell, I remember waking up with what felt like a full-blown hangover, even when I hadn't touched a drop of alcohol. It was the most bizarre and strange experience. I now learned that this was a result of Candida albicans in my gut fermenting the sugars from my diet, a form of 'auto-brewery', where they were producing acetaldehyde, a toxic by-product of ethanol (the substance that induces a hangover).

So here I was, being told the harsh truth that no student wants to hear – to quit sugar! I'd naively thought, up until then, that my diet was pretty well balanced. I was a pescatarian, I cooked most of my meals at university from scratch (a far cry from some of my flatmates' ready meals) and I tried to consume fruits and vegetables on a daily basis. In hindsight, I can see that I was still eating a very Westernised diet: three nights a week, I would tuck into my cheesy homemade lasagne for dinner with a meat substitute, served with a touch of lettuce and followed by a microwavable chocolate melt-in-the-middle pudding. Lunches would often consist of a tuna-mayo sandwich, crisps and a cereal bar, and breakfasts might be a sugary granola with milk and some strawberries. Let's not also forget the number of alcoholic beverages I would knock back on those big student nights out (think rum and Coke, Smirnoff Ice or vodka Red Bull).

But now I had to refrain from all forms of sugar (refined and natural – so that included fruit) and I was told that the stricter I was, the quicker my recovery would be. I initially took the news with a pinch of salt, while also considering the aesthetic benefits, wondering how much weight I might lose. But the more I thought about it, the more I felt compelled to follow the diet – because, honestly, what other option did I have? And anyway, it would be six weeks maximum, I thought, and then I'd be fighting fit, returning to my old student-life ways.

Begrudgingly, I followed the plan, propelled by the desire to start feeling better. I remember the first morning I started the diet, waking up to what looked like a bland breakfast of boiled egg, rocket and tomatoes. I had gone from carb overload to an extreme makeover of leafy greens overnight. My tastebuds were most definitely not impressed, and I couldn't wait for the next six weeks to be over.

Little did I know then that this would just be a first small step in my recovery. I had absolutely no idea about the life-changing journey that lay ahead of me.

Impacts of the illness

With the diet under way, I was counting down the days until the six weeks were up. Yet, as the weeks slipped by and my symptoms barely improved, I was devastated to be told to keep going with the diet. It was the most frustrating feeling in the world. One part of me contemplated quitting (it was clearly sacrificing my happiness), while the other considered the sinister prospect of living with this chronic illness for the rest of my life. I specifically remember my naturopath telling me at this time: 'There are people in this world who bounce back quickly to full health, and there are those who don't. Those who don't,' he said, 'are the people who should never give up and will value their health and the lessons learned more than anybody else one day.' Ten years have passed since then, and I can now say that he was right.

It is hard to put pen to paper when it comes to writing about my illness. At the time, I felt like I just existed. I was here, but I was not here. It was almost like an out-of-body experience. The severe brain fog was a surreal haze sweeping over me, making me feel continuously drunk and uncoordinated. I lost all concept of time, as my life – my golden years of youth – seemed to slip away from me.

And just like my life, the illness itself was not clearly defined. It was not like a virus that comes and then goes, just as quickly. I was living with it continuously, day in, day out, for years. There were good days, of course, and then there were bad days, but the condition was always lurking, a constant reminder to me to observe my limits, preventing me from living my life to the full.

The hardest part was the psychological toll. The thought that life would always be 'tinged' with this fatigue and mental haze was overwhelming and incredibly scary. But I was not prepared to live like that for ever. That's why I threw everything into the naturopathic regime.

As a student, all I wanted was to meet new people and go out and party. Instead, I had to go on nights out sober and I always felt like the boring one, even though I wanted to join in just like everybody else. It suppressed my personality in a way.

People would ask, 'Are you feeling better yet?' And I would feel shame and embarrassment having to confess that no, I wasn't. It wasn't long before some friends started to say negative things behind my back. I wanted them to understand, but perhaps it was wrong of me to expect them to. I should have just asked for their acceptance.

In the holidays, I would see friends for an hour, then need to go home and sleep. I wanted to simply sleep away the next few years, until it would all be over. The more I slept, the quicker the days passed. And this felt like a good thing – because it seemed to be taking me closer to my goal of recovery.

One of the hardest things to deal with at this point was the relationships that ended for me. I became really hung up on people not wanting to see me anymore and talking about me behind my back because I wasn't the 'fun Lauren' they used to know. I became fixated on this, naturally associating it with my illness. It was as though my illness became my identity; it really did change my whole world.

I felt like people didn't want to know me anymore because they saw me as boring, sick or because I couldn't socialise in the way that I was expected to (i.e. drink alcohol). I just didn't feel understood. Just because I looked healthy on the outside (my skin was great and I had lost some weight) did not mean that I felt that way on the inside. I was mobile, yes. I could get out of the house, yes. But that didn't mean that everything was ok, and it just reinforces the notion that people can be closed-minded when it comes to invisible illnesses. If they can't see something, then it doesn't exist to them.

Only my closest family knew the true extent of how I was affected daily. And truth be told, I realise now that I focused way too much on what I had lost than on the amazing people who were still there supporting me, like my family and those few friends who stood by me.

Food reactions

As a result of my illness, I developed a range of food reactions. This was during a period following the sugar-free regime, when I thought I would be able to reintroduce more foods into my diet – but after experimenting, I was surprised to learn that I couldn't tolerate certain things.

I became reactive to more and more different foods. Nothing I ate sat well, and I would leave the table after meals feeling absolutely terrible, with severe bloating, gas and digestive discomfort. There was a period when I was having regular colonics in a bid to make myself feel better – that's how bad it was.

I was told that I might have something called 'leaky gut' (where the cells lining the digestive system become permeable, enabling pathogens and food proteins to filter into the bloodstream, where they should not be). This is believed to trigger widespread symptoms, such as those I was experiencing with CFS, so I decided to take measures to tackle it.

I embarked on a gluten- and dairy-free diet, then eventually switched to a paleo diet (based on foods that people in the past could access by hunting and gathering). I drank bone broth (rich in glutamine, an amino acid known to promote the healing of intestinal cells) and incorporated prebiotic foods (such as Jerusalem artichokes, raw asparagus, onions and garlic) and probiotic foods (such as sauerkraut and kefir) to encourage a microflora balance within my gut.

My relationship with food

With all these dietary manoeuvres, people were starting to treat me differently, which was making me feel quite isolated. Food was all around me, and people saying, 'Let's catch up for a drink' or, 'Let's go out for dinner' made my stomach churn with anxiety. I would feel a frog in my throat as I attempted to explain about my health problems and what I was currently doing to try to beat them. Sometimes I just didn't want to get into it, but the topic was unavoidable, and I felt like I was always being scrutinised for it. It was *always* the bottom line: anything I did, everywhere I went, I was obsessing about food. It was the most exhausting thing in the world, and it felt like all the freedom and spontaneity had been taken out of life. Food ruled my mindset, and an intense fear of it became embedded within me.

Being anxious around food can create a catch-22 situation: if your body is in a state of stress while eating certain foods due to your fear of them, then, of course, symptoms (particularly digestive issues) can arise as a result. The first step in this particular battle was acknowledging that I had this problem, and I have since worked on rebuilding my relationship with food.

Ⓘ

A waiting game

I started to look at my illness through an entirely different lens, approaching it from many angles, peeling away the layers – like an onion – to try to get to the bottom of it.

The process of using alternative therapies can be immensely daunting and time-consuming (not to mention expensive – see also 'Recovery on a Budget', p. 299). I would do functional tests, which would often take time to be delivered to my flat, followed by waiting for delivery to the laboratory and then weeks of waiting for results to come through and then be interpreted by my practitioner.

I eagerly anticipated every consultation, phone call and email, desperate to find out if my digestive tract was clear of the pathogenic microbes I believed were driving my symptoms. But no matter how hard I worked on my diet, refraining from certain foods (while also supplementing with anti-microbial herbs), the process was agonisingly slow, and it felt like half the battle was just waiting – waiting for the day when it would all be over.

As months turned into years of working with natural-health practitioners, I slowly but surely improved, becoming more in tune with my body and how I was feeling. My gastrointestinal symptoms, along with several others, had largely improved (my intestinal flora were more in balance, with the help of some fantastic probiotic supplements I discovered). But my worst symptom – the overwhelming brain fog – still hung around.

As I worked with my naturopath on my diet and supplementation regime, he stressed that I needed to change not only my dietary habits, but also, ultimately, my whole lifestyle.

Lifestyle changes

We need to support our detoxification systems, monitor our stress and activity levels, get adequate rest and ensure that we are in the right frame of mind throughout the day in order to optimise wellness and recovery from illness. And this is where naturopathy comes into its own.

It may sound silly but having the right people around us is crucial as well. Being surrounded by 'toxic' people can be so damaging – so as well as eradicating unhealthy foods and toxic chemicals in our homes, we also need to detox our lives of unhealthy relationships, emotions, thoughts and behaviours.

In addition to all this, I also began to embrace rest and pace my activity levels, while practising meditation, yoga and breathing techniques that left me feeling calm and relaxed throughout the day, supporting me in dealing with stress and any bad days or setbacks with my health.

I started to become fully aware of my actions and behaviours. When my body sped up and I noticed that I was talking really fast, I would sense the need to slow myself down and remain in control.

Mindfulness – being aware of your behaviours and bringing yourself into the 'now' – is also incredibly important in all aspects of life.

Whether you are talking, going about your daily routine or eating, it is important to become aware of your thoughts and attitudes and remain in the present moment, in control of the task at hand, rather than distracting yourself with thoughts of the past or the future.

Eventually, I began to feel positive and optimistic about the future. Fortunately, I managed to complete my degree with a 2:1. It was a struggle, but I got there, having been granted some extensions on certain assignment deadlines due to my circumstances.

I started to wonder about my career path. In part, this made me anxious, as I questioned whether I could handle the working world because of the state of my health. Yet one of the most important things I had discovered was that I needed to do something that made me happy.

I decided that if I steeped myself in the industry of wellness and nutrition, it would be easier for me to maintain my self-care and ensure that I was in the best position to recover my health. So – largely motivated by my need to know more and get over chronic illness for once and for all – I enrolled in a nutrition and naturopathy course in London. This, I reasoned, would also allow me to use my personal experience to help others facing similar battles with their health. I wanted to turn my stumbling block into a stepping stone. And that's just what I did!

NLP: a flash course in optimism

Neuro-linguistic programming (NLP – more of which on pp. 263–276) is a form of self-development training that provides people with some very special and important skills, especially those who have become stuck in their lives or are experiencing problems with their health. It examines the interaction between mind and body, considering whether something has happened to halt a person's natural healing cycle and what has got in the way of the body trying naturally to recover. NLP then works on how people can coach themselves, enabling the brain to support the body in a more useful way.

NLP focuses very heavily on our language, thoughts (those which are quite often subconscious) and neurology, and how we can change our thoughts to change our health. Learning to become optimistic and adopt a positive outlook on any improvement – no matter how small – and celebrating all the good in your life are key to recovery. Poor health teaches us the importance of all the good in our lives.

Taking on board a more spiritual and philosophical approach to life has really broadened my perspective in combatting CFS, and I would absolutely recommend NLP to anybody struggling with chronic illness.

NLP really helped me in healing my relationship with food. I gained the confidence and ability to introduce more foods back into my diet and conquer a lot of the anxiety I had acquired around eating over the years, allowing me to find more of a balance and be less fear-driven. It also helped me with energy issues. I became more aware of when my body was slipping into 'fight-or-flight' mode (a stress response of the nervous system) and was able to work on calming anxious feelings, both to enhance energy and reduce anxiety, which ruled a lot of digestive and cognitive symptoms for me.

The mind is so powerful!

Where I am today

I have worked on reclaiming my mind and body from defeat, focusing on my health and fitness – something I have become truly passionate about – in the process. In April 2018, I even ran the London Marathon in celebration of having overcome so many obstacles with my health.

Going paleo, gluten-free, dairy-free, elimination diets, gut-healing protocols, colonics, detoxes, NLP, pacing, supplementation – you name it, I've done it. And while I don't believe that there's a one-size-fits-all when it comes to CFS, and there is no one magic bullet, the journey I went on has led me to where I am today, having regained my health.

Ten years on, and I am proud to have gained some valuable qualifications – a Bachelor of Arts in English Literature, diplomas in nutritional therapy and naturopathy, as well as in NLP, eating disorders and obesity. Alongside all this, I have also managed, as a result of my experience, to build a business – ARDERE – and I'm not shy about saying I'm really proud of that. Through ARDERE (pronounced ar-deh-ray, meaning 'glow'), my sister, Nicole, and I have teamed up to shine a light on healthy living. At ARDERE, we offer a 360-degree approach to wellbeing, from providing natural, effective and honest self-care products (including skincare), designed to enhance wellbeing, to the ARDERE wellness clinic, with nutrition, naturopathy and psychology specialists. You will find plenty of health resources on our website, ARDERE.com, too. We even have a customised recipe filter, where you can freely view nutritious recipes according to your dietary requirements (ideal if you are embarking on an elimination diet or have allergies or intolerances). Whether through following one of our healthy recipes, simply lighting an ARDERE candle in a bid to relax or using our natural skincare products, we want people to feel good in mind, body and soul.

Alternative therapies and lifestyle changes saved me, shaping me into the person I am today. They got me to follow a healthier path and to learn that health truly does begin with the lifestyle you lead. Naturopathy is a fantastic tool for uncovering information about why our bodies manifest symptoms that doctors cannot fathom. It equips us with the tools to prevent illness and support our health for the rest of our lives.

My future goals and aspirations

My goals for the future are exciting. I want to use my story to share my experience of CFS and tell others that there is hope out there; there are alternative therapies and lifestyle changes that can support the body's healing abilities, so that you can get your health back on track and improve your situation.

So now, without further ado, let's get to work.

PART 2
The Science

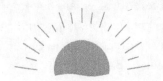

A reminder about pausing

I have made every effort to keep the science here as accessible and digestible as possible. So, while this section may require some patience, I'd encourage you to persevere, as it is more than worth the investment. Take your time with it, using the pause function, as mentioned earlier, to allow you to rest and digest when required and rereading where necessary to equip yourself with the information to help you better understand your own unique body, its physiological systems and the dysregulations that have been shown to be at play in CFS.

CHAPTER 2

CFS: What We Know So Far

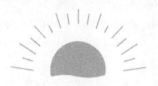

Knowledge is power.
Sir Francis Bacon, English philosopher and scientist

The subject of CFS is an ever-evolving narrative and, as such, it can be hugely controversial. Even as this book goes to press, there will no doubt be new emerging evidence, as we learn more about this complex condition.

While some professionals do not believe that CFS even exists, those who *do* accept its basis as a condition tend to argue as to whether it is physical or psychological in nature. Fortunately, in the last decade, professionals have been moving towards an understanding that CFS *is* a physical condition, although there is still some disagreement as to its origins.

I am going to provide you with as much clarity as possible, via a deep dive into everything you need to know about CFS, including the proposed causes, the implicated systems and the main symptoms.

A medical mystery: what is CFS?

CFS is a complex, chronic illness that profoundly affects the lives of those who experience it. It affects multiple body systems, including the nervous, neuroendocrine, immune and digestive systems, with evidence that there is a dysregulation between them, helping to explain the complex picture of symptoms seen in the illness.

What's in a name?

The terms CFS and ME (myalgic encephalomyelitis) are, as mentioned previously, often used interchangeably. But let's take a closer look at ME, starting with a breakdown of its name:

- My = a shortened form of *myo*, which means muscle
- Algic = the adjective form of *algia*, which means pain
- Encephalo = brain
- Myel = spinal cord
- Itis = inflammation

So ME refers to muscle pain and inflammation of the brain and spinal cord, and the term was introduced by the *Lancet* in the context of one of the first ME/CFS outbreaks, at the Royal Free Hospital in London, back in 1955. In fact, 'myalgic encephalomyelitis' is not a pathologically proven explanation for what happens in the body with this condition, but somehow we are still left with this long and confusing name.

Around thirty years later, ME was given another label – chronic fatigue syndrome (CFS), a term that caused significant outrage within the patient community because it was thought to trivialise their level of suffering. I would be inclined to agree.

It is a little like saying that somebody with Alzheimer's disease has chronic forgetfulness syndrome – it completely devalues the debilitating nature of the patient's experience.

The illness was also defined as 'yuppie flu' in the 1980s, making it sound like a fashionable form of hypochondria, due to its prevalence among twenty- to forty-year-old professionals.

In 2015, the US Institute of Medicine (now called The National Academy of Medicine) called for the condition to be known as systemic exertion-intolerance disease (SEID), further fuelling the confusion around how we should define it. And other terms such as post-viral fatigue syndrome, adrenal fatigue and burnout are also rife in this arena. No wonder people can get so confused!

Importantly, some healthcare professionals do categorise ME as a separate illness to CFS, although the vast majority of diagnostic criteria consider the two to be synonymous. As I said previously, I will use the term CFS throughout this book, despite my qualms about it, since it is the most widely used in medical literature right now.

Classifying CFS

How should we refer to CFS? Is it a syndrome? A disease? A disorder? An illness? A condition?

A syndrome refers to a constellation of signs or symptoms. The word comes from the Greek '*sundromos*', which means 'running together'. Symptoms may not always be 100 per cent consistent between patients and can also change over time, without always having an identifiable cause.

A disease is usually classified as a health condition with a clearly defined biological cause and a consistent change in anatomy, and a disorder is often used as a synonym for the word disease, although it more directly refers to an impairment in bodily structure or function (be it physical or mental). An example is an arrhythmia (an irregular heartbeat), which is a heart disorder that can stem from a known disease such as cardiovascular disease. Just to confuse things further, the word disorder is often used interchangeably with the word dysfunction.

An illness is a broader, more woolly term, which is subjective and refers to a person's feelings or experience that may (or may not) occur from a disease. This might be pain, fatigue, weakness, nausea and can be influenced by disease factors, as well as non-disease factors such as beliefs, fears, mood and your environment.

A condition is indicative of a person's state of overall health. Again, it is another broad term that can refer to all the above, and even non-pathological situations, such as pregnancy or childbirth. It is essentially the status of a person, based upon their functional capacities and their positioning on a spectrum of illness to wellness.

The correct terminology for CFS is still much debated in the medical world, but for the purposes of this book I will interchangeably use the words condition, dysfunction, disorder, illness and syndrome to refer to CFS.

How CFS manifests

CFS tends to adopt a fluctuating relapsing and remitting pattern, which can look different from one sufferer to the next.

While there is some diversity in the symptoms themselves, too, the one that is broadly shared by the majority of CFS patients is called post-exertional malaise (PEM), which I refer to as 'payback'.

Symptoms of CFS are seemingly endless, but common ones include:

- Fatigue
- Post-exertional malaise (PEM or 'payback')
- Cognitive impairment, including brain fog, memory problems and lapses in concentration
- Painful muscles and joints (myalgia)
- Gastrointestinal symptoms, such as those common in IBS (indigestion, bloating, gas, diarrhoea or constipation)
- Stress-related symptoms (anxiety, panic and difficulty tolerating stress)
- Food and alcohol intolerance
- Increased sensitivity to chemicals, smells, temperatures, sounds

or light
- Heart palpitations
- Vertigo or dizziness
- Nausea
- Orthostatic intolerance (where symptoms become worse upon standing)
- Repeated flu-like symptoms (malaise, fever, recurrent sore throat)

Note: you do not need to have all the above symptoms to have CFS (see 'The diagnosis dilemma', p. 31).

Post-exertional malaise (PEM)

PEM refers to the feeling of fatigue or other CFS symptoms worsening following any form of exercise, activity or exertion. Somebody struggling with PEM may feel much worse and crash with fatigue after walking to their local shops or even to the other end of their garden. In severe cases, sufferers can experience PEM from minor tasks, such as taking a shower or even brushing their teeth. It can also arise from mental exertion or stressful experiences; it's like a form of payback from previous activities. Importantly, the fatigue experienced by sufferers is incredibly debilitating and life-impacting.

PEM remains one of the hallmark symptoms that distinguishes CFS from other overlapping conditions, such as depression. In depression, exercise has been shown to improve patient outcomes, whereas CFS patients tend to get much worse with exercise.

Who is affected by CFS?

Epidemiologists at the CDC (Centers for Disease Control and Prevention) in the US estimate that CFS affects 17–24 million people worldwide. (Epidemiologists can be defined as disease detectives who study how often illnesses occur in groups of people.) In the UK, CFS has been shown to affect 250,000 people; however, problems with diagnosing the illness, as well as the surge in those suffering with long COVID, which shares some association with CFS (see pp. 33–34), could mean that the number is a lot higher in reality.

CFS has been found in twice as many women as men and can affect any social class, ethnicity and age group, including children and adolescents.

There are two peak times when CFS is known to occur in particular – during teenage years and early adulthood. However, it does not discriminate against any age group.

A spectrum disorder: sub-types of CFS

CFS is a spectrum disorder, which means that everyone is affected in totally different ways.

- **Mild:** those who are mobile and still in work or education

- **Moderate:** those with reduced mobility who have likely stopped work or education, or have had to make adjustments, such as working part-time

- **Severe:** those who are house/wheelchair/bed-bound and may have difficulty with speech and swallowing. In some very severe situations, patients are tube-fed and highly sensitive to light and sound. Severe cases are known to affect 25 per cent of the total CFS population.

A study in the journal *PLoS One* found that when compared with twenty different conditions (including rheumatoid arthritis, stroke, lung cancer and schizophrenia), patients with CFS reported the lowest health-related quality of life.[1]

A 2019 study in the *Occupational Medicine* journal explored the work status of 508 CFS patients,[2] reporting that 55 per cent were working, 16 per cent were temporarily taking leave and 29 per cent had stopped working altogether.

It is therefore clear to see that the illness has a detrimental impact on jobs and livelihoods, with many sufferers putting their careers on pause and seeking health benefits to support themselves financially.

The diagnosis dilemma

Because of the long list of symptoms experienced in CFS (see p. 28), which can mimic those of many other diseases, doctors must first rule out alternative medical possibilities before a final diagnosis of CFS can be made. Therefore, CFS is a diagnosis of exclusion because:

- there are no standard medical tests for diagnosing the illness
- cases vary and there is no one consistent set of symptoms.

Some argue that CFS is a 'dustbin diagnosis' – a label for your symptoms but no solid answers to explain them. However, the National Institute for Health and Care Excellence (NICE – the UK's go-to guidance system within the NHS) sets out a protocol for healthcare professionals whereby, once standard GP investigations and testing have ruled out other illnesses, a CFS diagnosis is made when the following symptoms have persisted for at least three months:

- Debilitating fatigue that is worsened by activity and is not relieved by rest.

- Post-exertional malaise in which the worsening of symptoms:
  - is often delayed in onset by hours or days
  - is disproportionate to the activity

    – has a prolonged recovery time that may last hours, days, weeks
    or longer.

- Unrefreshing sleep or sleep disturbance (or both), which may include:
  – feeling exhausted, flu-like and stiff upon waking
  – broken or shallow sleep, altered sleep pattern or hypersomnia.

- Cognitive difficulties (often described as 'brain fog'), which
  can include problems finding words or numbers, slowed
  responsiveness, difficulty speaking, short-term memory problems
  and trouble concentrating or multi-tasking.[3]

Note: while the above are the main symptoms required for a CFS
diagnosis in the UK, the diagnostic criteria can vary across the world. I
have listed the many other symptoms that can be present in CFS on p. 28.

It is clearly a problem that patients must wait a minimum of three
months before getting the answers they need and an accurate diagnosis. However, with a complex array of symptoms, varying diagnostic
criteria around the world and the absence of a hard medical test, it is
certainly a challenge for healthcare professionals to diagnose this illness
promptly without the need to rule out other illnesses first. This is the
diagnosis dilemma.

Co-morbidities

A co-morbidity is when a medical condition occurs alongside another.
One of the reasons why CFS is so controversial is because the cluster of
symptoms that characterise the illness can overlap with various other
conditions. It also doesn't help that the symptoms of CFS are often
vague and non-specific.

Let's take, for example, the symptom of fatigue. This is a highly subjective symptom, which means it has different connotations for different
people. Fatigue has been linked with conditions such as depression,
anxiety, cancer, sleep disorders, fibromyalgia, Lyme disease, autoimmune and thyroid diseases, among many others.

Then we have digestive symptoms, which include bloating, flatulence and abdominal pain. These are all very common in CFS, yet they do not appear on the list of key symptoms in most criteria for diagnosing the illness. These symptoms overlap with irritable bowel syndrome (IBS), coeliac disease and inflammatory-bowel disorders, such as Crohn's disease or ulcerative colitis, which also need to be ruled out by a process of elimination.

Other conditions that can commonly exist in combination with CFS include Ehlers-Danlos syndrome (a group of connective-tissue disorders) and postural orthostatic tachycardia syndrome (PoTS).

Problems with diagnosis

There is clearly a long way to go in correctly diagnosing CFS. Up to 80 per cent of sufferers can go undiagnosed,[4] and therefore the patient population is under-reported in the medical literature.

I am a case in point. I requested a copy of my medical records over the last ten years while writing this book; however, I could not find any *official* diagnosis of CFS on file, despite my doctors having said that CFS was what I was struggling with.

Also, while many CFS sufferers go undiagnosed by the medical community, there are other people who are *incorrectly* diagnosed with CFS. Two UK surveys[5] have revealed that 49 per cent of patients referred to a specialist CFS clinic had alternative medical diagnoses upon further investigation. Some of these included sleep disorders and depression, which introduces more ambiguity into this complex diagnostic arena.

Long COVID and CFS

Since the COVID-19 pandemic, the worldwide medical system has seen huge surges of chronically unwell patients reporting ongoing symptoms following an (often mild) SARS-CoV-2 infection. With a symptomology that is much akin to that of CFS, this is currently being defined as long COVID (not to be confused with post-intensive-care syndrome, which refers to patients who are experiencing long-term complications, such as respiratory, cardiac problems or organ damage, after being hospitalised with COVID-19). Over £20 million of research has been pledged by the National Institute for Health and Care Research (NIHR) to tackle long COVID, which, due to the similarities, could shine a light on our understanding of CFS in the future, too.

An invisible illness

It is common for some patients with CFS to be met with disbelief by their doctor, and, in some cases, professionals blame symptoms on psychological factors instead. This is an example of medical gaslighting.

One reason for the lack of understanding around CFS is that you cannot see this illness – it is invisible. In recent years, however, society has made huge strides in its collective understanding of mental-health concerns, such as depression and anxiety, and this acceptance must now also extend towards other invisible illnesses, like CFS.

Treatment for CFS

Unfortunately, there is no proven medical cure for CFS. However, management interventions have been implemented by the healthcare system to support patients with symptoms.

The interventions that have been historically put in place include:

- graded exercise therapy (GET)
- cognitive behavioural therapy (CBT)[6]
- medication(s) to manage symptoms such as pain, nausea or sleeping problems.

Graded exercise therapy (GET)

GET is a structured exercise programme that aims to gradually increase your physical activity levels and usually involves exercises that increase heart rate, such as walking or swimming. Once activity levels have been established, a healthcare professional will work to set goals to increase the intensity and duration of exercise moving forwards. This happens irrespective of patient feedback, even if they feel worse following exercise.

This therapy gained momentum because of a 2011 study funded by the UK Medical Research Council, called the PACE trial. Conducted on 641 patients, PACE was one of the largest randomised trials for CFS, examining interventions such as CBT and GET. Results were published in the *Lancet*, suggesting that a full recovery from CFS was possible following these interventions, so justifying the NHS's recommendation for CBT and GET for patients.

However, the PACE trial and, in particular, GET have faced harsh criticism from patients, clinicians, researchers and CFS charities alike, following numerous reports that GET was making patients' CFS much worse. An independent survey[7] of CFS patients was commissioned by Forward-ME in 2019, to feed into the NICE guideline review process, which found that 81 per cent of patients' symptoms worsened after receiving GET. One of the criticisms is that physical activity is increased regardless of how the patient is feeling, often ignoring an increase in (or onset of new) symptoms.

Note: distinct from GET, another way of incorporating activity is called grading, which we will discuss in detail on p. 225. This involves increasing your activity and maintaining it for a period before attempting another increase. A key difference between grading and GET is that the targets are not so rigidly applied. It is a slow, gentle and steady approach to recovery that does not put strain on the nervous system or ignore increasing symptoms that arise along the way (post-exertional malaise), allowing patients to listen to their bodies (and not to anyone else). Activity should be increased marginally and only when the body is willing.

Cognitive behavioural therapy (CBT)

CBT is a form of talking therapy that works to support changes in the way people think and behave. It is used in the management of anxiety, depression, eating disorders and IBS, as well as CFS. CBT is based on the concept that your thoughts, feelings, physical sensations and actions are all interconnected, and that negative ways of thinking keep you trapped in a vicious cycle.

In a CBT session, you work with a therapist to break down your problems into parts, such as thoughts, physical feelings and actions, establishing whether they are helpful or unhelpful to you, and considering steps that may be necessary to change them.

There is some conflicting data when it comes to CBT and patient outcomes in CFS. Some patients have reported a worsening of their symptoms following CBT, whereas others have experienced little change or a significant improvement in symptoms. Some experts think that for those who experience a worsening of their condition following CBT it may be because they feel that their illness is being psychologised. I would be inclined to agree. I often find that when CFS patients understand that their condition is physical but can be supported by psychological therapies, CBT can provide numerous benefits to their health.

CBT and GET: where we are now

The theory behind using CBT and GET to treat CFS was based upon the view that the condition is caused by patients feeling tired and unwell because of inactivity and deconditioning, as well as holding negative illness beliefs. This clearly fails to account for the fact that the illness is physical, the implication being that simply moving more and thinking more positively is the way to go. Unfortunately, the reality is that you cannot force your way out of this illness through physical activity and it can, in fact, often do more harm than good.

As a result of the PACE trial having been discredited among the research community, as well as thousands of patients complaining of worsening symptoms following GET, NICE updated their guidelines in

2021, moving away from recommending GET as a therapy for CFS. This is a fantastic step forward.

NICE guidelines have also reframed recommendations around CBT and CFS, simply citing it as a *management* tool for the psychological effects of chronic illness, as opposed to a curative therapy for CFS.

Medication

There is no specific medicine for CFS. However, there are medicines that can help to relieve symptoms. Over-the-counter painkillers can be used to ease headaches and muscle and joint pain, while some GPs might prescribe antidepressants for those with chronic pain or trouble sleeping.

What causes CFS?

Currently, we do not know precisely what causes CFS. However, emerging evidence is starting to provide some fascinating insights about the factors at play.

CFS has a three-pronged structure, broken down into three Ps:

- Predisposition
- Precipitating trigger(s)
- Perpetuating factor(s)

Predisposition	Precipitating trigger(s)	Perpetuating factor(s)
Genetics	Infectious agent (viral/bacterial/parasitic), surgery, trauma, stress, toxic exposure, vaccination	Dysregulation and chronic stressors (deficiencies and/or toxicities)

Predisposition

It is widely believed that CFS has a genetic component. In 2001, a twin study[8] examined concordance rates related to CFS (a concordance rate is a term used to describe the percentage probability that two people with shared genes will develop the same disease). The study found that the concordance rate was significantly higher in identical than in non-identical twins. This indicates that disease risk may be increased due to genetic rather than environmental factors.

What's more, in early 2020 a large Norwegian genetic study discovered that two versions of genes (called alleles) were linked with CFS.[9] These alleles are part of the HLA (human leukocyte antigens) gene family, which make proteins essential for the immune system to recognise different pathogens and have been linked with autoimmune diseases. Scientists found that these were more common in CFS patients than in healthy people – a finding that points towards problems with the immune system in CFS, which we will explore later (see p. 57).

In 2020, a research grant was awarded for further study into CFS and any genetic links. A collaboration of researchers, people with CFS, carers and advocates, the Decode ME study is being led by the ME/CFS Biomedical Partnership and is currently searching for DNA features that may make someone more (or less) likely to become unwell with CFS.[10] This will hopefully uncover more clues as to the genetic causes of the illness as we progress in our understanding of CFS.

Precipitating trigger(s)

One thing that *is* clear in the scientific literature is that a trigger episode often causes the onset of the CFS.

An investigation into the precipitating factors of CFS showed:[11]

- 72 per cent of patients reported an infectious illness upon becoming unwell (for more on infectious agents linked with CFS, see pp. 57–58)
- 28 per cent of patients had no apparent infectious trigger, but instead reported a traumatic event (such as a car accident or a fall) or surgery
- stressful life events were also reported to be very common in the year preceding the illness.

In my clinical experience, approximately 90 per cent of the CFS patients who come to see me report having had a recent infection (mostly viral, but in some cases bacterial or parasitic). You can clearly see how the term post-viral fatigue syndrome was coined!

However, CFS onset does not always follow in the wake of an infection. I have also had clients come to see me having become unwell after a recent surgery.

I have also seen people who had glandular fever in childhood, then, years later, they experienced a significant traumatic and stressful event and then boom – CFS hit. Others have been asymptomatic carriers of infection and thereafter struck down with CFS. And there have also been reports of CFS occurring after vaccination,[12] breast-implant surgery [13] and exposure to chemical toxins.[14]

These are all classic examples of a 'haven't-been-well-since . . .' scenario. (See also the tipping-point diagram on p. 92.)

Perpetuating factor(s)

As well as predispositions and precipitating triggers towards developing CFS, there are other factors that can perpetuate symptoms. Left unaddressed, these can stop patients from moving forwards in their recovery.

These perpetuating factors include:

* dysregulated systems (see diagram on p. 41)
* chronic stressors (also known as deficiencies and/or toxicities, see p. 79).

These, and their role in CFS, will be covered in more detail in the chapters that follow.

Pathophysiology

Pathophysiology is a fancy term referring to the physiological processes in the body that are affected in an illness.

We are going to explore the pathophysiology of CFS, uncovering the physical and biomedical roots of what is happening within the body to perpetuate the various fatigue-related symptoms experienced by patients, so dismantling the notion that CFS is a psychological condition.

CFS is a dysfunction affecting multiple bodily systems. Therefore, there isn't one specific part of the body to focus all our attention on or blame; it is a disorder in the way that the body *functions* and operates on a day-to-day basis.

It's a software, not a hardware problem

When you first go to your doctor with a health concern, they will conduct some basic medical tests. They might request an X-ray or CT scan, for example.

In this sense, doctors are looking at all the basic *hardware* to see if they can identify any structural issues.

However, standard medical testing does not dive much deeper than certain conventional markers, and if you have CFS it is very likely that all your medical tests will come back normal.

We need to view this illness as a *software* – or 'physiological systems' – problem, but conventional healthcare offers a reductionist approach, often approaching each part of the body and each system as a separate entity in isolation, rather than looking at the whole. Take, for example cardiologists, who study the heart, and ophthalmologists, who are specialists in the eyes. This compartmentalised perspective fails to consider how the body is one intricately interconnected system, which is particularly important when we are dealing with CFS.

It is only through very detailed research into the deeper systems of the body that we are starting to unravel the clinical clues as to what is happening in people with CFS. This sets the stage for what I am going to discuss next, which is called 'physiological dysregulation'.

Physiological dysregulation

The term 'physiology' refers to the branch of biology relating to the function of bodily systems, and how these processes work to respond to daily challenges.

Every time you breathe, open your eyes, digest your food, regulate your sleep cycle or take a step, physiological processes are at play. You can also face additional internal demands when you encounter injury or an infection. And on top of this, the body must also respond to external demands, typically related to environment – exposure to pollen or pollution or changes in gravity and temperature, for example. All these call for the various systems of the body to be working hard to allow you to perform specific functions.

But how is all this relevant?

Well, emerging evidence indicates that in CFS, these physiological processes can become dysregulated, explaining the various symptoms experienced in the illness. The diagram below lists the complex web of dysregulations that have been shown to occur within CFS:

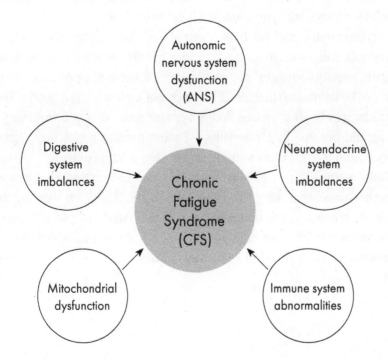

Dysregulated systems

In a healthy human body, physiological feedback systems work in a tightly controlled manner to handle the various demands outlined above efficiently. This is a form of balance, known as homeostasis.

However, in CFS, the body's systems are thought to become imbalanced, such that the body becomes unable to handle basic daily demands. These disruptions in physiological mechanisms are referred to as *dysregulation*.

As seen in the diagram on the previous page, the physiological systems dealing with our daily demands typically include:

- the autonomic nervous system (ANS)
- the neuroendocrine system
- the immune system
- the mitochondria
- the digestive system.

These systems all communicate with and somewhat depend on one another to work efficiently. When they become dysregulated in CFS, the body throws out symptoms as a form of feedback.

Post-exertional malaise is an example of this because the body is physically communicating that it cannot handle the level of physical or mental activity demanded of it and is saying it needs to ease off and rest.

It can be helpful to think of CFS in terms of having a 'noisy' body. The disturbances in your various bodily systems mean that you feel everything and become highly sensitive. I often explain it this way to my clients, and it helps them to understand what is happening.

Daily demands can heavily feed into the CFS symptom picture, whether those that are placed upon the body at a given moment in time or, indeed, in the hours and days beforehand. To put it simply, a person with CFS has a highly sensitised set of systems, which means they cannot effectively deal with daily demands.

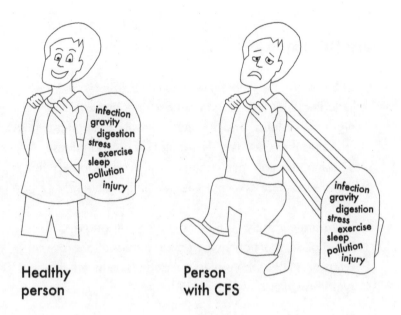

**Healthy
person**

**Person
with CFS**

As you can see in the illustration above, the healthy person is able to carry their backpack and handle daily demands without a problem. The person with CFS, on the other hand, has several dysregulated systems and is therefore challenged by the various demands placed upon them, driving symptoms further.

Let's imagine that the healthy person has had a poor night's sleep. On top of this, he is having a difficult time due to worrying about an upcoming exam. So he might feel a little stressed and tired today, but, because his systems are working optimally, he will likely feel perfectly fine and energised again tomorrow.

For a person with CFS, it doesn't quite work in the same way. A poor night's sleep compounded by a stressful day can add fuel to the fire of their illness, causing alterations in their physiological systems and therefore prompting flares and crashes of their symptoms. I've had clients in the past refer to the illness as like 'walking through treacle', and this is certainly the case when patients experience this 'flip-flopping' scenario.

In the coming chapters, we will look in more detail at dysregulated systems and the medical hypotheses that have been used to explain CFS.

Key takeaways

- CFS is a chronic illness that affects multiple bodily systems, including the nervous, neuroendocrine, immune and digestive systems, and the mitochondria. Emerging evidence indicates that there is a dysregulation between these dynamic physiological systems, which helps to explain the complex picture of symptoms seen in the illness.

- There are currently no medical tests to diagnose CFS. Diagnosis occurs only when other explanations for your symptoms have been ruled out and if you match the symptom criteria on pp. 31–32.

- Scientists do not know what causes CFS; however, mounting evidence points towards genetic links (predisposition), precipitating trigger episodes (such as infections, surgery, vaccinations and trauma) and perpetuating factors (dysregulated systems and chronic stressors).

- There is currently no medical cure for CFS.

CHAPTER 3

The Nervous System

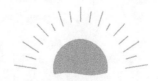

Calmness is the cradle of power.
Josiah Gilbert Holland, American novelist and poet

The nervous system is a major controlling and regulatory system. It communicates with various parts of the body to govern mental activities and physical movement, as well as the unconscious actions we do daily.

It transmits electrical signals (known as nerve impulses) between different parts of the body and can be divided up into the central and peripheral nervous systems (see the diagram on the next page). The central nervous system encompasses the brain and spinal cord, whereas the peripheral nervous system connects the central nervous system to the rest of the body, via tiny cable-like fibres called nerves.

The peripheral nervous system can be subdivided into the somatic nervous system and the autonomic nervous system (ANS). We will be focusing on the ANS.

Autonomic nervous system (ANS)

The ANS is the involuntary branch of the nervous system, controlling our breathing, heart rate, body temperature and digestion. It is also involved in the functioning of the body's organs, muscles and glands.

The ANS can be divided as follows:

- The sympathetic nervous system (SNS)
- The parasympathetic nervous system (PNS)
- The enteric nervous system (ENS)

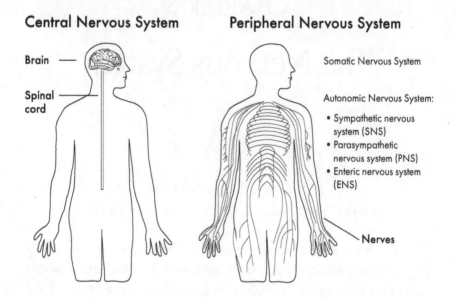

Central Nervous System

Brain

Spinal cord

Peripheral Nervous System

Somatic Nervous System

Autonomic Nervous System:
- Sympathetic nervous system (SNS)
- Parasympathetic nervous system (PNS)
- Enteric nervous system (ENS)

Nerves

We will talk about the ENS a bit later (see p. 71), but for now, let's keep our attention on the SNS and PNS.

Also referred to as the body's 'fight-or-flight' response, the SNS is activated when the body is primed for action to run away from physical danger. Evolutionarily speaking, when we were cavemen, back in the day, our fight-or-flight response was essential for our survival when we were being chased by that sabre-toothed tiger. The SNS response ensures that we quickly get away from a threat. Blood is pumped to our muscles, our heart rate and blood pressure rise, while adrenaline and noradrenaline (two of the body's major stress hormones) are secreted into the bloodstream.

Fortunately, nowadays we are unlikely to experience sabre-toothed-tiger attacks, but instead we face other stressors (exams, for example, or job interviews), and our bodies respond to these in much the same way, using the fight-or-flight response.

The parasympathetic nervous system (PNS), on the other hand, talks you down from danger (it basically undoes the work of the SNS after a stressful situation). Also referred to as our 'rest-and-digest' response, it is the normal functioning state that the body operates in when it is relaxed and rested. It slows breathing and heart rate, constricts pupils and encourages digestion. Living in our stressful, modern-day world, this is the state that we could all do with spending most of our time in.

AUTONOMIC NERVOUS SYSTEM

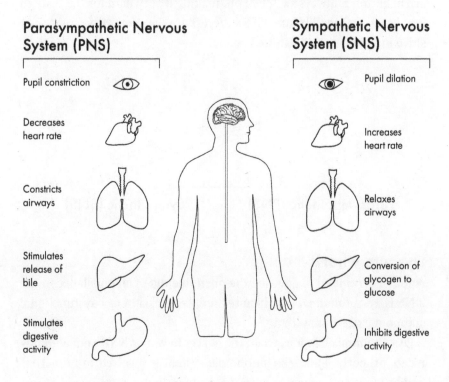

Parasympathetic Nervous System (PNS)

Pupil constriction

Decreases heart rate

Constricts airways

Stimulates release of bile

Stimulates digestive activity

Sympathetic Nervous System (SNS)

Pupil dilation

Increases heart rate

Relaxes airways

Conversion of glycogen to glucose

Inhibits digestive activity

The ANS is able to switch from PNS to SNS mode, depending on what external signals the body experiences. The body can only ever be in one of these states at a given moment in time; therefore the SNS and PNS are much like yin and yang – stress vs relaxation or panic vs peace.

But how does all this link to CFS, I hear you ask? Bear with me, I'm getting there!

ANS dysfunction in CFS

Mountains of scientific research papers show nervous-system involvement in CFS,[15] with some convincing evidence pointing towards the body being chronically tipped into SNS mode, out of its natural sync or harmony with the PNS.

This is called SNS predominance, which means that the body has become wired towards operating in a stressed-out state. The stress-alarm button is always switched on, making it very hard for the body to find its natural equilibrium. CFS sufferers are therefore very stress-sensitive individuals, as illustrated below.

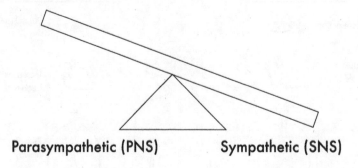

Parasympathetic (PNS)   Sympathetic (SNS)

Dysauto-what?!

Another term used to describe the phenomenon of an imbalance in the ANS is dysautonomia, which quite literally translates to a dysfunctional autonomic nervous system.

Dysautonomia happens when the nerves in your ANS do not communicate properly. Since the autonomic system is involved in numerous bodily functions, when it starts to malfunction you are prone to experiencing a variety of symptoms as a result. These include:

- fatigue
- insomnia
- heart palpitations
- orthostatic intolerance (being unable to stand up for long periods of time without feeling dizzy or light-headed)
- brain fog, concentration and memory problems

- increased sensitivity to chemicals, smells, temperatures, sounds or light
- cold hands and feet
- nausea
- pain
- anxiety and/or difficulties tolerating stress
- irritable bowel and bladder symptoms.

Still with me? I hope so!

In Part 3 (p. 93), you will learn some key strategies for supporting the health of your nervous system and improving activation of the PNS.

Key takeaways

- The ANS forms part of the peripheral nervous system, and incorporates the body's central response to stress (known as the SNS, aka 'fight-or-flight' response) and relaxation (known as the PNS or 'rest-and-digest' mode) and the enteric nervous system (ENS).

- Evidence indicates that in CFS, the body is tipped into SNS mode (also known as SNS predominance), meaning the body is in an ongoing state of stress.

- Dysautonomia is another term for when the ANS is out of balance and malfunctions, causing a number of the characteristic symptoms of CFS.

Now let's move on to another part of the body that has been discovered to be affected in CFS: the neuroendocrine system.

CHAPTER 4

The Neuroendocrine System

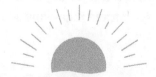

Don't judge each day by the harvest you reap,
but by the seeds that you plant.
Robert Louis Stevenson, Scottish novelist

Let's start by breaking down the word 'neuroendocrine':

- Neuro – relating to the brain and nervous system

- Endocrine – relating to our hormones (chemical messengers that transmit information, regulate important metabolic processes and work to control the interaction between the body's organs and cells) and glands (organs throughout the body that secrete hormones)

The neuroendocrine system is a network of glands and organs where the nervous and endocrine systems interact. It's how the brain regulates hormonal activity in the body.

Importantly, this involves a part of the brain called the hypothalamus, which secretes hormones and controls homeostasis (a state of balance). The pituitary gland is like the hypothalamus's little brother, positioned just below it and operating under its control. The size of a pea, it stores and secretes hormones produced by the hypothalamus, as well as synthesising some of its own.

There are five key components – or axes – in the neuroendocrine system. These axes refer to the way in which hormones are released from the hypothalamus and pituitary to action specific functions in different parts of the body:

- HPA axis (hypothalamic–pituitary–adrenal axis)
- HPT axis (hypothalamic–pituitary–thyroid axis)
- HPG axis (hypothalamic–pituitary–gonadal axis)
- HPP axis (hypothalamic–pituitary–prolactin axis)
- HPS axis (hypothalamic-pituitary-somatotropic axis)

You could think of the neuroendocrine system as being a bit like an orchestra, whereby if one player is out of tune the entire performance is compromised. The HPA and the HPT axes are a big focus in CFS, as we will see.

The HPA axis

The HPA axis involves an intimate relationship between the hypothalamus, pituitary and adrenal glands, and is best known for conducting the body's response to stress in the immediate minutes following the activation of the sympathetic nervous system (SNS).

When something stressful happens, the body's immediate response comes from the SNS (see p. 46). A few minutes later, the HPA axis kicks in, as the hypothalamus responds to the surge of adrenaline and noradrenaline by releasing corticotropin-releasing hormone (CRH) into the bloodstream.

CRH perpetuates the effects of the SNS response, such as a raised heart rate and pupil dilation. In addition, it tells the pituitary gland to secrete adrenocorticotropic hormone (ACTH) into the bloodstream. ACTH travels down to the adrenal glands (these are two tiny grape-sized glands above the kidneys), where it prompts the release of cortisol from the adrenal outer layer (known as the cortex).

Cortisol

Cortisol is one of the body's major stress hormones; it is a steroid that follows a circadian rhythm, usually peaking within thirty to forty minutes after we wake up and gradually decreasing to its lowest point at night. Stress has been shown to cause an increased cortisol output; and when stress becomes chronic, it causes sustained activation of the HPA axis.

The release of cortisol incites several physiological changes that help the body to deal with stress:

- It mobilises sugars like glucose into the blood.
- It increases blood pressure.
- It inhibits processes deemed of lesser importance during a stressful event. Examples include the suppression of reproductive activities, digestion and immune function.

While these changes are indeed helpful in the short term, they can pose health troubles in the long term if the stress response is not regulated.

The HPA axis and CFS

It's clear that some hormonal disturbances occur in CFS. Since the HPA axis is heavily involved in our bodies' longer-term response to stress, tiredness is a likely result when this becomes out of whack. Scientific literature suggests that there is suppression of the HPA axis with a low output of adrenal hormones[16, 17](known as adrenal insufficiency) in CFS patients.

In a healthy individual, receptors in the brain sense when a stressor has passed and shut off the stress response through what is known as a negative-feedback loop. However, this loop can become impaired, resulting in the ongoing high production of cortisol and adrenaline.

Adrenal insufficiency can therefore occur because of chronically high cortisol levels and a perpetual stress response, with the adrenals eventually tiring out. It's like your adrenal glands have had enough of it, so they start to sleep. When this happens, their output starts to reduce, meaning the body is far less able to tolerate stress and perform optimal bodily functions. This is something I see time and time again with clients and have first-hand experience of myself.

This can help to explain the various symptoms involved in CFS, including fatigue, brain fog, blood-sugar problems, impaired stress tolerance, aches, pains and also insomnia.

Adrenal Fatigue: Fact or Fiction?

The term 'adrenal fatigue' tends to go hand in hand with adrenal insufficiency and applies to a collection of non-specific symptoms, much like CFS (fatigue, aches and pains, sleep problems and digestive troubles).

It happens when the adrenal glands are unable to keep up with the demands of a perpetual stress response. As a result, the HPA axis slows down and the adrenals cannot produce enough of the right hormones for the body to stay healthy. This may be because the body has been predominantly firing a fight-or-flight state.

It is not an accepted medical diagnosis, per se, but this doesn't mean to say it is not a reality.

Note: this is not to be confused with Addison's disease, an autoimmune condition which causes complete failure of the adrenal glands to secrete the hormone cortisol.

The HPT axis

The HPT axis involves the hypothalamus, pituitary and thyroid glands and primarily functions to maintain normal circulating levels of thyroid hormones.

The thyroid gland

The thyroid is a butterfly-shaped gland situated at the base of the neck, just below the Adam's apple. It is responsible for secreting several different hormones that work to control our metabolism, growth, development and body temperature.

The most notable thyroid hormones include:

- Thyroxine (T4)
- Triiodothyronine (T3)

T4 is the inactive form of thyroid hormone, which gets converted in the body to T3 (the biologically active form). These hormones are produced by the thyroid gland when the pituitary releases something called thyroid-stimulating hormone (TSH).

The thyroid governs a lot of energy-demanding processes and has fingers in various bodily pies that control metabolism and daily functioning. Therefore it should come as no surprise that, when the thyroid is out of kilter, symptoms much like those in CFS can arise: fatigue, brain fog, memory problems, headaches, low blood sugar, digestive issues and pain.

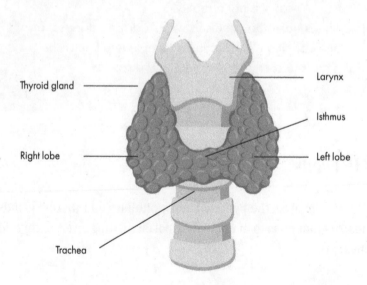

Hypo- and hyperthyroidism

It is possible for the thyroid gland to under-function (known as hypothyroidism, where it does not produce enough thyroid hormones) or become overactive (hyperthyroidism, where it produces too many thyroid hormones).

One of the confusing things here is that fatigue and other CFS-related symptoms can arise from both hypo- and hyperthyroidism. In addition, there are autoimmune conditions that can cause hypo- and hyperthyroidism. These include:

- Hashimoto's thyroiditis (when the immune system produces antibodies that attack the thyroid gland, causing a failure to produce sufficient thyroid hormones)

- Grave's disease (when the immune system attacks the thyroid gland, causing it to make more thyroid hormones than the body needs).

That's why it is so important for thyroid disease to be initially ruled out prior to a diagnosis of CFS being made.

What's the thyroid doing in CFS?

Lower levels of thyroid hormones appear to be evident in studies on CFS patients, in the absence of a hard diagnosis of thyroidal disease. This was shown in a 2018 investigation,[18] examining ninety-eight CFS patients against ninety-nine healthy ones. The results uncovered normal levels of TSH in those with CFS (which was also the case in the healthy patients); however, CFS patients were found to have lower blood levels of T3 and T4 than healthy controls.

The HPT axis and CFS

While a hard diagnosis of hypo- or hyperthyroidism may not be discoverable from a standard NHS blood test, it might still be the case that some underlying thyroid dysfunction is driving symptoms in some CFS patients.

In Part 3, we will cover how to balance adrenal and thyroid hormones, why it is important to have your thyroid fully investigated in CFS and some of the functional tests available for this (see pp. 113–118).

Key takeaways

- The neuroendocrine system is where the hypothalamus and pituitary gland interact with the body to release hormones.

- During times of stress, the HPA axis kicks in straight after the SNS response by releasing cortisol.

- In CFS, adrenal insufficiency can occur through suppression of the HPA axis.

- The thyroid releases hormones that support energy-demanding processes. It is possible for the thyroid to become underactive (hypothyroidism) or overactive (hyperthyroidism).

- In CFS, thyroid insufficiency can occur even in the absence of a hard thyroid disease (which is why functional testing has its value).

CHAPTER 5

The Immune System

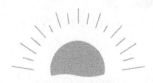

It is health that is real wealth, and not pieces of gold or silver.
Mahatma Gandhi, Indian lawyer,
nationalist and political ethicist

The immune system is made up of specialised cells, organs and chemicals that work to fight infection and keep our bodies healthy. As such, it is incredibly intelligent.

Infections occur when microorganisms (whether bacteria, viruses, fungi or parasites) enter the body, multiply and cause illness, as the body reacts to the invading microbe(s).

What's happening with the immune system in CFS?

Scientific literature is still investigating how the immune system behaves in CFS but, for simplicity, we should consider what I call 'the three Is':

- Infection(s)
- Inflammation
- Immune dysfunction

Infections and CFS

Infections associated with triggering the onset of CFS include:

Viral:
- Herpes viruses (for example, Epstein–Barr – aka glandular fever – cytomegalovirus, human herpes virus 6 (HHV-6), varicella-zoster)
- Enteroviruses (for example, coxsackievirus)
- Parvovirus B19
- Dengue fever
- Ebola
- Hepatitis
- Ross River virus (Australia)
- SARS-CoV-2 (in the case of long COVID)

Bacterial:
- Coxiella burnetii (also known as Q fever)
- Chlamydia pneumoniae
- Mycoplasma
- Borrelia burgdorferi (causes Lyme disease)

Parasitic:
- Giardia
- Blastocystis hominis
- Dientamoeba fragilis

Chronic infection and CFS: waking the sleeping lions

Some patients with CFS experience an ongoing immune response, even after an infection has cleared, while others may suffer with a chronic infection that might be driving their symptoms (this is a popular theory among those investigating the causes of long COVID,[19] too).

After recovery from an initial bout of a viral infection, viruses can remain dormant – known as a latent infection. At certain life periods and in some individuals, latent infections can reactivate and contribute to ongoing symptoms. This is thought to occur in a subgroup of CFS patients.

Chronic infections associated with CFS include Borrelia burgdorferi, mycoplasma and human herpes viruses. Persistent infections can also be found in the gut, such as Candida albicans and parasites like Dientamoeba fragilis (see pp. 74–75).

Infections can occur either independently or, in some cases, together, when they are known as co-infections.

Chronic Lyme disease and CFS

Lyme disease is a bacterial infection caused by Borrelia burgdorferi, which is spread to people by infected ticks. Ticks can carry many other pathogens alongside Borrelia bacteria, including Bartonella, Babesia and Rickettsia (this is why ticks are often called 'dirty needles'). Ten to twenty per cent of Lyme disease cases can result in chronic symptoms that overlap with CFS (fatigue, brain fog and post-exertional malaise are all key features). This can happen when the initial infection is not spotted and left untreated (and even in some cases where treatment is given).

Many people refer to these ongoing symptoms as 'chronic Lyme disease'. Due to the striking resemblance between the two conditions, some experts argue that chronic Lyme disease is simply another term for CFS, triggered by the Borrelia bacteria.

Inflammation and CFS

The body has a whole host of responses to infection or injury. One of these is a process called inflammation, which happens when the immune system defends the body from things that would normally harm it, such as an infection or injury, sending white blood cells, redness, swelling, pain and heat to the area affected.

Inflammation is a crucial part of innate immunity. It is the immune system's response to an irritant (such as a germ or even a foreign object like a splinter in your finger).

But hold on . . . there is a catch!

Chronic inflammation

While inflammation is normal and essential and, in acute cases, like a cut on the leg or a short-term infection, it is not going to pose us too much trouble, the problem starts when it becomes chronic – when the body's immune system *continues* an inflammatory response, even after the threat has gone. And it can become damaging to the body's own tissues.

Inflammation should therefore be a closed loop; it should have a beginning, middle and, very importantly, an end – once the threat has been resolved. If the loop is left open, chronic inflammation results, and can last for months or even years.

Chronic inflammation has been linked to a variety of health conditions, such as obesity, type-2 diabetes and autoimmune conditions, such as rheumatoid arthritis.

Chronic inflammation in CFS: should we blame the infection or our bodies?

When you become unwell with an infection, it is not the pathogen that causes you to feel ill. It is your body's *response* to that microorganism that causes the classic symptoms of feeling unwell. You know, the feeling you get when you are coming down with something: tiredness, joint aches and a fever. This happens when the immune system releases its key army troops, such as cytokines, which are part of the inflammatory response to fight off infection.

Cytokines are small proteins released by cells (including immune cells) that coordinate the body's response to infection and trigger inflammation. When cytokines flood the body at a much higher rate than normal, it is known as a cytokine storm.

In CFS, cytokines are pro-inflammatory molecules that do not get properly switched off and can eventually cause damage to the body's own tissues (studies have found elevated levels in CFS patients, which may correlate to the severity of the person's illness[20]). Not only that, but pro-inflammatory cytokines (and chronic inflammation in general) are heavily linked to feelings of fatigue and malaise.

It is thought that part of the problem in CFS is that the immune system is being hypervigilant and simply doesn't know when to quit. Even after the acute trigger infection has gone, it is believed that, in some cases, the immune system generates an ongoing inflammatory reaction to the pathogen, making the sufferer chronically unwell.

Immune dysfunction and CFS

In CFS, as we've seen, the body's inflammatory response is simply not working in the best interests of our health. What's more, immune dysfunction can also happen through an immune response called auto-immunity.

Autoimmunity is essentially a case of mistaken identity, whereby the immune system attacks the body's own tissues instead of a foreign invader (also known as a loss of self-tolerance).

Fatigue and brain fog feature strongly in various autoimmune conditions, such as rheumatoid arthritis and lupus. Some of the literature surrounding CFS posits that the condition is autoimmune in nature, due to findings of raised autoantibody levels (antibodies that attack bodily tissues) in some of the CFS patient population.[21]

Some experts even believe that autoimmune activity might be a consequence of CFS, rather than a direct cause of it. It is suspected that in some cases, a triggering infection (or perhaps another agent, such as surgery or immunisation) can lead to processes that induce autoimmune responses (known as molecular mimicry and bystander activation).

CFS and autoimmunity: too early to say?

It is, perhaps, a little premature to conclude that CFS is an autoimmune condition as such because, while there are clusters of CFS patients expressing autoimmune activity in their bodies, there are others with no evidence of this.

This is where understanding the illness starts to get complex because we may be looking at different sub-types under the umbrella of CFS. Ultimately, what we do know is that an erratic immune response is at play, which might explain chronic inflammation and the reactivation of latent viruses in some CFS patients.

Mast-cell involvement

Growing evidence links problems with mast cells (regulators of the immune system found in every tissue in the body) and CFS (and long COVID) symptoms.

Mast cells play a big role in inflammatory and allergic responses and release over 1000 different chemical mediators, such as histamine. Mast-cell-activation syndrome (MCAS) occurs when the mast cells in the body release too many chemical mediators at the wrong times. The mast cells get excitable and are prone to blowing up in response to any form of stimulation, such as infections, stress and rapid temperature changes, as well as certain foods and chemicals.

Allergy and CFS

There is a significant link between allergies and CFS. An allergy is when the body has an adverse immune response to something ordinarily harmless (an allergen), such as food, pollen, dust or other substance to which it has become hypersensitive. Some allergies might be related to MCAS; however, they can also arise from other immune-mediated mechanisms, such as an antibody response (through an antibody called IgE).

Additionally, many CFS patients report problems when they are exposed to environmental chemicals, which is known as multiple chemical sensitivity (MCS), as well as suffering with food reactions. See Part 3 for more on food allergy, food intolerance and food sensitivity, along with diet and lifestyle measures you can take to support your immune system.

Key takeaways

- The immune system is thought to be involved in CFS via infection, inflammation and immune dysfunction.

- Some patients with CFS can experience an ongoing immune response, even after an infection has cleared, while others may suffer with a chronic infection that might be driving their symptoms.

- Studies have shown that chronic inflammation occurs in CFS patients, particularly through increased levels of cytokines (molecules heavily linked with fatigue).

- Immune dysfunction is also thought to occur in CFS through a process called autoimmunity, where the immune system attacks its own tissues.

CHAPTER 6

Mitochondria and Energy Metabolism

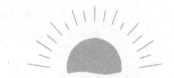

Where focus goes, energy flows.
Tony Robbins, American author

Our bodies are made up of different types of cells, such as muscle and nerve cells, and each of these requires energy to do its job. Cue the mitochondria: tiny bean-shaped structures inside each of our cells that produce energy for our physical and mental functioning – a bit like batteries.

Whether you want to scratch your head, climb the stairs or focus on your work, your mitochondria play a leading role in all these activities. Nicknamed the 'powerhouse of the cell', mitochondria get to work by breaking down food into energy through a process called cellular respiration. Whenever we eat carbohydrates, our mitochondria turn these sugars into fuel by creating a molecule called ATP (adenosine triphosphate) – our bodies' energy currency compound.

What are the mitochondria doing in CFS?

Since one of the main features of CFS is fatigue, disturbances in the mitochondria are an attractive explanation for scientists, given their major role in energy production. However, studies have confirmed that it is uncommon to see genetic mutations in patients' mitochondrial DNA, suggesting that CFS does not appear to be a mitochondrial disease.[22]

Nevertheless, while there may not be any *physical* problems with the mitochondria in CFS, mitochondrial dysfunction – whereby something is blocking their ability to produce energy – appears to be happening instead, and the science in support of this idea is gaining traction.

Mitochondrial dysfunction: an explanation for CFS symptoms

Researchers have discovered that CFS patients have decreased production of ATP, compared with healthy groups of people.[23,24]

When the mitochondria stop working properly, the resulting poor supply of ATP to the body's cells causes them to slow down because they don't have enough energy to function normally (where energy demand exceeds delivery), meaning that bodily functions start to slow down, too.

The processes that mitochondria play a role in include the following:

• Energy production
• Nerve impulses
• Muscle contractions
• Immune regulation
• Heat production
• Cell death (known as apoptosis) – this is particularly important when we are battling viral infections

Since the mitochondria are involved in these various bodily processes, mitochondrial dysfunction may help to explain particular CFS features, including fatigue, brain fog, muscle pain and flu-like symptoms.

Infections, inflammation, environmental toxins, oxidative stress, nutritional deficiencies and psychological stress can all cause mitochondrial dysfunction.

(II)

Deconditioning vs dysregulation

As well as their condition often being blamed on psychological causes, one of the other frustrations for many CFS sufferers is when their symptoms are blamed on deconditioning (changes in the body that occur due to a lack of physical activity, such as a loss of muscle size and strength). This is often seen in the elderly population who experience inactivity or long periods of bed rest due to illness. For many people with CFS, this implies that they are lazy and simply feel tired because they haven't exercised in a while.

However, as we have established, dysregulation of the body's main functional systems is the contributor towards CFS symptoms, not deconditioning. One argument for this is the symptom of post-exertional malaise (PEM – see p. 29), which has not been detected in deconditioned people. The research shows that PEM may be explained by dysregulation, particularly of the mitochondria.

This is thought to occur because energy demand exceeds energy delivery in CFS – i.e. the demand for ATP is higher than the mitochondria can supply. Mitochondria must be good at recycling ATP to keep the cells constantly topped up with energy. If they are impaired due to slow recycling, cells must shut down and wait until more ATP is made. This can take time – days, even – and explains why some people can take a long while to recover after experiencing PEM.

Importantly, one of the key differences between deconditioning and dysregulation is that deconditioning *improves* with exercise and is more easily reversed, whereas dysregulation is often worsened by it (involving an exaggerated response to normal levels of activity).

The deconditioning theory was one of the flawed justifications for the use of graded exercise therapy (GET), which, as we saw earlier (see pp. 35–36), has been scrapped as a treatment for CFS.

In Part 3, we will explore how to optimise mitochondrial function to enhance your energy.

Key takeaways

- The mitochondria are tiny bean-shaped structures inside our cells, which produce energy in the form of a molecule called ATP.

- Scientists have found that CFS patients have a lower production of ATP compared with healthy people.

- When there is not enough ATP supplied to the body's cells, our systems start to slow down as a result.

- Mitochondrial dysfunction is thought to be an explanation behind the symptom of post-exertional malaise (PEM) in CFS.

CHAPTER 7

The Digestive System

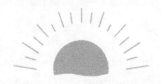

Gut health is the key to overall health.
Kris Carr, American author and wellness activist

Our digestive systems are critically important to overall health and longevity, so it should come as no surprise to learn that research is linking the health of the gut with various conditions, including CFS.

One study reported that 92 per cent of CFS patients experience irritable bowel syndrome (IBS).[25] In most cases, IBS symptoms precede the onset of CFS itself. IBS is known to affect 11 per cent of the world's population (and about one in five people in the UK). Common symptoms include bloating, abdominal pain, constipation and diarrhoea.

Because so many people with CFS also suffer with digestive concerns, it raises the question: is there a gut origin for CFS? Scientists are starting to uncover some fascinating clues about the role of the gut in CFS, even when digestive symptoms (such as IBS) are not overtly apparent.

'All disease begins in the gut'

So said Hippocrates, the father of modern medicine.

As we walk through the evidence to date linking the gut with some of the key body systems affected in CFS, this chapter will also cover the various gut imbalances that have been associated with the illness, including:

- dysbiosis
- infection(s)
- inflammation and intestinal permeability.

But first, let's introduce the inner world of the digestive system, known as the microbiome, establishing what it is and how it plays a pivotal role in our health.

What is the microbiome?

A whole world of microorganisms lives in and on the human body, and emerging science indicates just how important this is in terms of health and longevity. In fact, did you know that we are more bacteria than we are human? We have trillions – yes, trillions – of bacteria living on our skin, in our mouths and, of course, in our guts. (An estimated 500–1000 species live within our digestive tracts alone.[26])

The term microbiome has become something of a buzzword, referring to the communities of microbes (bacteria, fungi, viruses, protozoa and archaea) that reside within a particular environment – for example, the digestive system. It's a bit like a tropical rainforest, with all sorts of species living in the same habitat.

And what's more, your microbiome is much like a fingerprint in that it is entirely unique to you.

Note: the term microbiota is sometimes used interchangeably with microbiome, although there is a slight difference. Microbiome refers to the bugs *and* their genes (yes, bacteria and viruses have genes), so it incorporates the whole ecosystem, whereas the term microbiota refers solely to the microbes in a particular environment, for example, the gut. Some other terms that you might hear in this context include gut flora and microflora, which are used synonymously with the word microbiota.

The gut microbiome: a powerful player in our health

Your microbiome is constantly changing and can be influenced through lifestyle factors such as a nutritious diet, which is highly important for a diverse microbial ecosystem (we will come to this in Part 3).

As I've explained, there are various types of bacteria living in and on the body. However, most of these microbial residents are found in the gut. There is certainly some form of chatter going on between the bacterial communities in our guts and our various bodily systems, offering a plethora of benefits to our wellbeing.

While it might seem obvious that there is an important role for bacteria in gut health, the benefits of the microbiome are more far-reaching than simply supporting digestion. In fact, the microbiome is known to influence energy, digestion, immunity, the thyroid, metabolism, hormones, neurotransmitters, mitochondria and even our detoxification capacities. Gut bacteria have even been shown to regulate our gene expression, too.

What's more, certain types of bacteria can help the body to absorb particular nutrients from our diets (such as iron and magnesium), as well as producing and synthesising others like vitamin K, B12 and folate. Gut bacteria also regulate glucose and fat metabolism, which can play a role in preventing chronic diseases such as type-2 diabetes and obesity.

The gut: where bacteria and the immune system meet

The gut is the first place where our internal worlds come into contact with our surrounding environments, via the food and drink we ingest, which means it plays an important role in protecting us against any pathogens that go down the hatch.

Once food and drink have travelled down the oesophagus, stomach acid helps with digestion, as well as neutralising any bacteria that may cause illness or food poisoning. Following contact with the stomach, foods or liquids then pass into the small intestine, where they meet the richest density of immune cells in the body (impressively, the gut is the body's largest immune organ). The small intestine is also the site where most of our nutrient absorption takes place.

The gut wall also houses the gut's most abundant antibody, called secretory immunoglobulin A (SIgA), which has anti-inflammatory properties and is secreted in vast amounts in the gut to bind and eliminate toxins and pathogens to wash them out of the body. We secrete grams and grams of this antibody every single day.

Our gut microbes educate the immune system to distinguish between what is harmful and what is our own tissue, preventing autoimmune responses and ensuring overall wellbeing.

When things start to go wrong with this relationship and the body is exposed to factors that reduce the diversity of bugs in the microbiome (for example, a poor diet, antibiotics, infections, stress, heavy metals, pesticides and moulds), this can snowball into impaired immunity, which occurs in CFS.

Where the gut and the nervous system meet: the gut-brain axis

Ever heard anyone tell you to 'listen to your gut'? Well, this stems from the fascinating connection between the belly and brain, known as the gut–brain axis.

The gut–brain axis is a bi-directional communication pathway between the nerves in the digestive tract and the central nervous system (CNS). The lining of the gut contains more than 100 million neurons called the enteric nervous system (ENS), which forms part of our autonomic nervous system (ANS).

While the brain sends signals to the ENS, the ENS communicates messages back to the brain such that both the CNS and ENS inform, control and respond to each other's signals.

A key interface for the gut and brain to connect is through the vagus nerve, one of the longest cranial nerves, running from the brain stem right down into the abdomen. The vagus nerve acts as a walkie-talkie, controlling parasympathetic activity in the body, and our gut microbes love to use it as a conduit to talk to the brain. There have been studies associating a poorly functioning vagus nerve with some of the cognitive symptoms (such as brain fog) seen in CFS.[27]

The gut–brain axis also highlights why you may feel digestive symptoms because of stress or nervousness. Whenever you feel the urge to use the bathroom ahead of a big exam or you have butterflies in your tummy before a big interview, that's your gut–brain talking!

Our microbiome and the mitochondria

While science has popularised the term gut–brain axis, we are also coming to understand the unique intricacies between the microbiome and the mitochondria (our cells' energy batteries – see p. 64).

Did you know that mitochondria evolved from ancient bacteria over 1 billion years ago? In fact, our mitochondria and gut bacteria form a close relationship where the gut microbiome influences all the mitochondria in the human body. Mitochondria rely on the bacteria in the gut to provide them with the nutrients (metabolites) they need to function. These are called short-chain fatty acids (SCFAs) and serve as fuel for the mitochondria; they also support the generation of new mitochondria in our cells.

All these little aspects of our cellular health are connected when it comes to dealing with CFS.

The gut and the thyroid

Healthy functioning of the thyroid gland is dependent upon intestinal bacteria, which produce an enzyme called intestinal sulfatase. Intestinal sulfatase supports the conversion of the inactive T4 thyroid hormone into the active T3 hormone, which plays a pivotal role in energy levels. Twenty per cent of this conversion happens in the gut, and that's why it's so important to take care of your gut health. If you have an unhealthy microbiome, the chances are that you'll have poor thyroid hormone conversion, too.

Classification of gut bacteria

You may have heard talk of 'good' and 'bad' bacteria. Unfortunately, however, it is not as straightforward as this.

While there are various species of bacteria in the gut that perform a multitude of roles, it is true that some can be considered as more 'disruptive' than others that are more beneficial to our health.

When it comes to the more beneficial bacteria, there are two types of symbiotic (close and long-term) relationships at play here:

- Mutualism: where both the microbe and human benefit and thrive
- Commensalism: where one benefits and the other is unaffected

To add confusion, most of the beneficial bacteria in the gut have a mutualistic relationship with us humans – however, we typically refer to these as our 'commensal' bacteria. These friendly commensals need to be kept within a delicate balance because, if circumstances allow and they overgrow or become deficient, they can wreak havoc, causing problems for our health, known as dysbiosis.

At this point you are probably thinking, why is this relevant to CFS? Trust me, I'm getting there; I'm simply setting the stage . . .

Dysbiosis: the role of microbes in CFS

The term dysbiosis simply refers to an imbalance in the microorganisms in the gut. Dysbiosis can involve:

- a deficiency of commensal organisms
- an overgrowth of commensal organisms
- an overgrowth of disruptive or pathogenic microbes
- an overgrowth of microbes in the wrong place: for example, the small intestine (known as small intestinal bacterial overgrowth, or SIBO)
- low diversity of commensal organisms.

Sometimes, dysbiosis can involve a combination of these factors.

Many studies have found dysbiosis in the microbiomes of CFS patients.[28,29,30] This includes reduced diversity of bacteria in the gut, with lower numbers of Bifidobacteria (which is also starting to ring true of long-COVID patients). Bifidobacteria have been shown to keep the immune system in check and maintain gut-barrier integrity, so it is no surprise that lower levels may be contributing to the compromised immune systems and gut linings seen in CFS patients.

More than 90 per cent of human diseases are linked with microbiome dysbiosis, including allergies, anxiety, Crohn's disease, coeliac disease, eczema, diabetes, depression and rheumatoid arthritis, as well as CFS, of course.

Dysbiosis can be caused by various lifestyle factors (including antibiotics, stress, a poor diet and toxic chemicals). In Part 3, we will uncover ways to maintain a healthy balance of bacteria in the gut when recovering from CFS.

Candida albicans

Candida is a type of fungus (yeast) that is naturally present in the gut, mouth, skin and vagina.

Ordinarily, a healthy human body contains a good balance of candida, which forms part of the mycobiome (the fungal communities living in and on the body). However, a species called Candida albicans is opportunistic and can overgrow, causing health problems (including vaginal thrush), as well as widespread symptoms such as fatigue, brain fog, bloating, diarrhoea, constipation, food and chemical intolerances and sugar cravings. The picture of symptoms for a candida infection is, as you can see, similar to that of CFS.

Candida infections can be driven by high-sugar diets or weakened immunity, as well as some medications (such as antibiotics or the oral contraceptive pill). It is possible to test for yeast infections via a comprehensive stool test, which can detect the presence of fungal overgrowth. I often do this with my clients in clinic.

When I was unwell, there was a point at which candida was blamed as the sole culprit for everything I was going through. However, as I have come to understand the microbiome (and the rest of the body) on a much deeper level, I believe that pointing the finger in this way is naive. Yes, Candida albicans might form *part* of the dysbiosis and infection picture in *some* CFS cases, but it's just one piece of a very complex puzzle.

Parasites

Parasites are organisms that live off hosts to survive. Some do not affect their hosts, whereas others can grow and reproduce to make people sick. Parasitic infections linked with CFS include Giardia, Blastocystis hominis and Dientamoeba fragilis.

What's more, parasites can steal nutrients from your diet for their own selfish gain, leading to nutritional deficiencies, which can further impair cellular and physiological health.

Viruses in the gut

If you were fascinated to learn that we are more bacteria than human, you may also be surprised to learn that we are, in fact, more virus than we are bacteria!

The body is host to many different viruses (known collectively as the virome) and, just like bacteria, some can cause disease, whereas others are completely harmless or even potentially beneficial. It is estimated that up to 380 trillion viruses are harboured in the human body.

The gut contains the most abundant population of viruses compared with other areas of the body. Most gut viruses are known as bacteriophages; these can live in and on bacteria, changing their genetic material and killing them.

It is becoming clear that dysbiosis of the gut is commonplace in CFS, particularly due to the reduced diversity of gut bacteria species. Since viruses can affect the populations of gut bacteria, researchers are now asking the question, is dysbiosis in CFS somehow connected to changes in the gut virome?

Gut inflammation: joining the dots in fatigue

So how does this all link with fatigue? Well, this is where our old friend inflammation rears its ugly head once again.

Dysbiosis can incite inflammatory processes within the gut and compromise the integrity of the gut lining, which can lead to a leaky gut (also known as intestinal permeability). Leaky gut happens when undigested food particles, bacteria and toxins seep through the gut wall into the bloodstream, inciting an inflammatory surge (this can set the stage for autoimmune disease). Some degree of leaky gut is a natural phenomenon in the human body, but problems arise when gut permeability becomes chronic, contributing to the inflammatory cascade that is common in CFS.

Drivers of leaky gut include dysbiosis, chronic inflammation, chronic infections (for example, viruses, parasites, candida) and lifestyle factors such as stress, medications, a poor diet, excessive alcohol intake and environmental toxins.

When you start to understand the relationship between the health of your gut and immune and nervous systems, it becomes easy to see how an imbalanced gut and inflammation can contribute to poor health. And it makes sense that if the gut is disturbed, physical and mental fatigue can follow because of the inflammatory response, which is associated with feelings of tiredness and malaise. Inflammation and leaky gut can also impair our ability to absorb nutrients, making us more susceptible to developing nutritional deficiencies and food sensitivities, both of which are common in CFS.

There is some controversy among healthcare professionals as to whether leaky gut is a cause of CFS or a secondary symptom (known as an epiphenomenon) running alongside the illness. However, a robust gut lining is important in bolstering your body's defences against inflammation – which is why we will be uncovering ways to restore gut health through dietary and lifestyle approaches in Part 3.

Key takeaways

- The gut supports the health of various other parts of the body, including the nervous system, thyroid, immune system and mitochondria.

- The gut is thought to be involved in CFS through dysbiosis, infection and chronic inflammation.

- The gut microbiome refers to the community of microorganisms (for example, bacteria, viruses, parasites and fungi) that reside within the digestive system.

- Dysbiosis refers to an imbalance of microorganisms in the gut, which has been shown to occur in CFS.

- Gut infections linked with CFS include parasites, Candida albicans and viruses.

- Dysbiosis and infections in CFS can cause leaky gut, which sets the stage for chronic inflammation.

CHAPTER 8

Chronic Stressors: Deficiencies and Toxicities

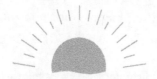

It is more important to know what sort of person has a disease than to know what sort of disease a person has.
Hippocrates, Greek physician

We have discussed the various dysregulations that have been shown to be at play and what the research shows so far in CFS. It is my belief that these malfunctioning systems become a source of stress in the body, driving a self-perpetuating vicious cycle of symptoms following a trigger event (for example, an infection, surgery, vaccination or trauma).

Therefore, fatigue and the sea of all-consuming symptoms in CFS are an alarm system communicating that something is not quite right within the body and needs addressing. In this way, CFS can be viewed as a chronic physiological response to a storm of threats, compounded by a multitude of ongoing stressors.

These chronic stressors can be grouped into 'deficiencies' and 'toxicities':

Deficiencies	Toxicities
Adrenal insufficiency (HPA axis dysfunction)	Infections, inflammation, dysbiosis and immune dysregulation
Thyroid insufficiency	SNS predominance (ANS dysfunction)
Mitochondrial insufficiency	Environmental toxins, allergies and oxidative stress
Nutritional deficiency (for example, CoQ10, carnitine, B vitamins, iron, antioxidants)	Stress and trauma

- **Deficiencies** refer to the inadequacies of hormonal functioning in CFS patients (such as the adrenals and thyroid gland), combined with low mitochondrial output and nutritional deficiencies.

- **Toxicities** may include the presence of infections, dysbiosis, immune disturbances and inflammation. They also include ANS dysfunction, where the body is chronically geared towards SNS (fight-or-flight) mode. Toxicities may also refer to physical or psychological stress, allergies and oxidative stress, as well as environmental overloads, such as toxic exposure to heavy metals, pesticides or moulds.

In combination, these deficiencies and toxicities can be seen to perpetuate symptoms of illness because they incite poor cellular and physiological health. Moreover, these stressors can also feed into one another, forming the complexity of the illness. For example, environmental toxins, infections, stress, nutritional deficiencies and oxidative stress can impair mitochondrial function; stress and SNS predominance can contribute to adrenal insufficiency; while dysbiosis, inflammation, environmental toxins and nutritional deficiencies can also drive low thyroid output.

So there are numerous tensions occurring here, where one stressor pulls on another and compounds the body's dysregulations, perpetuating CFS symptoms and impeding recovery. Some CFS patients might have only one or two of these imbalances, whereas others may require support in several different areas on the deficiencies and toxicities list.

In Part 3, we will cover how you can identify and address any underlying deficiencies and toxicities.

Tired or toxic?

A toxin can broadly be described as any substance that is harmful or poisonous to the body. Toxins can be external, from the environment, or alternatively they can be produced within the body, such as endotoxins produced by our gut bacteria.

Exposure to toxic chemicals has been implicated as a risk factor for many serious health conditions including cancer and neurological diseases, as well as the many autoimmune diseases and, of course, CFS.

We have identified that some people become unwell following toxic exposure as a *trigger* for CFS (such as farmers spraying agricultural chemicals and pesticides on their land), but it is also true that toxins can accumulate in the body over the course of an illness (and even *prior to* CFS onset), much like a drip effect.

Toxic exposure can, therefore, result in CFS instantaneously, through launching a cascade of immune responses and dysregulations as a trigger, or it can drive symptoms insidiously by impairing the cell structures that produce energy, such as the mitochondria. Toxins can also cause immune, endocrine and microbiome disturbances, as well as oxidative stress and ANS dysfunction. Toxic exposure is therefore a potential trigger *and* driver of CFS symptoms in some individuals.

The body's toxic soup

CFS patients tend to become more sensitive to toxins and synthetic chemicals within their environment. This is partially related to ANS and immune dysfunction, but also because the liver may have become overburdened and is struggling to detoxify these chemicals, which then start to accumulate in the body and cause illness.

There are three main ways toxins can get into the body:

- Ingestion – mainly through food and water
- Inhalation – breathing them in
- Via the skin – this happens through direct contact (for example, through clothing, applying substances to the skin or through the air or water)

Luckily, our bodies have developed sophisticated methods of removing unwanted, harmful toxins. The main detoxification organs include the liver, kidneys, lungs, skin, and gut, which work in concert with the circulatory and lymphatic systems.

Toxins associated with CFS

While there are too many toxic substances to list in this book, here are some of the key ones associated with CFS:

- **Heavy metals** These are elements that are naturally found within the earth and include mercury, lead, nickel, aluminium, cadmium, chromium and arsenic. Often used for various modern-day purposes, such as agriculture and medicine, they can also contribute to heavy-metal poisoning and have been linked with CFS.

- **Pesticides** Also known as organophosphates, pesticides are widely used on farms to spray crops and for use as sheep dips. They are also used in the garden for pest control and in the house for killing pet fleas. There have been many cases of farmers developing CFS; it has been linked to sheep dipping (with a lack of protective attire). Glyphosate is an example of an organophosphate compound (the best-known example of this is RoundUp), which can end up in the food supply.

- **Mould mycotoxins** Mould is a type of fungus that can grow and release toxins (known as mycotoxins) that can disrupt our physiology and fuel inflammation, leading to ill health, including immune-system problems. Many people can associate their CFS symptoms with being in a particular building (often termed 'sick-building syndrome') or environment – often old or damp and mouldy places with poor ventilation.

Other known environmental toxins include polychlorinated bi-phenyls (PCBs), bisphenols (such as BPA), as well as volatile organic compounds (VOCs), alcohol, tobacco smoke, food additives, fluoride, chlorine, phthalates, dioxins, heterocyclic amines, nitrosamines, PFAS, triclosan and EMFs.

Stress and trauma

Many of my clients are wary of discussing stress because it throws up concerns that the illness is 'all in their heads'. While I completely acknowledge that the illness is physical, stress and trauma are chronic stressors that can disrupt the body's physiology and drive the various symptoms we see in CFS. Stress simply *adds* to the load of dysregulations that form the picture of this illness.

But what is stress? And how does it differ from trauma?

Stress is a state of strain or tension resulting from adverse or demanding circumstances. It is a response to demands that require either a physical or emotional adjustment. Stress can therefore be physical or psychological and it is a way for our bodies to tackle threats to our wellbeing (whether real or perceived).

Trauma is a stressful experience that activates a robust emotional response. Traumatic experiences are always stressful, but stressful experiences are not always traumatic.

It is also important to know that some stress (known as acute stress) is good for us, helping us to perform under pressure and acting as a motivating force (for example, doing exams or working towards a deadline). Chronic stress, however, is not so great (see p. 86).

Psychological sources of stress include:

- pressures at work or in education
- relationship difficulties
- financial concerns
- health problems
- the death of a loved one
- a traumatic event such as a natural disaster, rape or theft.

Note: even happy events can cause stress in our lives – for example, planning a wedding, moving house or a pregnancy.

Physical sources of stress include:

- a poor diet
- smoking
- high alcohol consumption
- lack of/disturbed sleep
- stimulants (caffeine, blue light, technology exposure)
- environmental toxins
- chronic infections
- gut problems (including food intolerances and sensitivities).

We can further categorise stress into micro- and macro-stressors:

Micro-stressors: small common stress triggers that happen on a daily basis	Macro-stressors: life-impacting events or experiences that cause an overwhelming amount of stress
Your alarm did not go off and you are late for your doctor's appointment	A chronic illness
A bad night's sleep	Losing your job or facing financial difficulty
Skipping lunch	Death of a loved one
Getting stuck in traffic	Being bullied, neglected or experiencing sexual/domestic abuse
An argument with someone	Adverse childhood experiences (ACEs)
An untidy house	Relationship breakdown (divorce or family rifts)
Having to cancel a commitment due to a crash in chronic-illness symptoms	Witnessing a violent crime or natural disaster
Seeing bad news on the television	Car accident or fall

Generally, we have some level of control over micro-stressors and can influence our ability to deal with them, but we often have less control over macro-stressors, and they can place a large burden on our health.

It is the macro-stressors that tend to be experienced as trauma. Of course, trauma is highly subjective and what one person finds traumatic, another may not. (And the same goes for micro-stressors.) You might think you don't have trauma in your life (such as severe grief or an adverse life event), but trauma can be anything that you *perceive* as traumatic.

You will also notice that having a chronic illness can be classed as a macro-stressor and for many people, this is experienced as trauma. Chronic illness can cause people to grieve their losses, such as the life they had before they were unwell (for example, a job, financial stability, fulfilment and great relationships). Often, these are the things largely affected in chronic illness, and so it is not surprising that many people with CFS find their illness traumatic.

Adverse childhood experiences (ACEs) and CFS

ACEs are, as the name suggests, stressful and potentially traumatic events that occur in childhood. Examples include bullying, racism, parents separating, physical, sexual or emotional abuse, witnessing violence, the death of a caregiver or substance abuse in the family.

What many people do not realise is that childhood sets the stage for how we deal with stress over the course of our lives, impacting our resilience, hard-wiring the body for stress. In fact, studies have discovered that you are six times more likely to develop CFS if you have had ACEs.[31]

What's in your stress bucket?

The stresses we are faced with – both psychological and physical – all go into our stress buckets.

Have a think about your current situation and the history of stress in your life leading up to this point. In the table below, tick the stressors that are applicable to you and cross off those that are not:

Stressor	✔	X
Poor diet		
Working long hours without much time to rest (before CFS)		
Relationship breakdown		
Regularly skipping meals		
Death of a loved one		
Smoking		
History of abuse or bullying		
High alcohol/caffeine intake		
History of ACEs		
Gut problems		
History of ill health (for example, frequent infections, prior diagnosis such as IBS)		
Lack of sleep		
Exposure to environmental toxins (for example, working in agriculture, construction, nail salon, hairdresser, aerospace and flight crew)		
Frequent use of medications (for example, antibiotics or NSAIDs)		
Intense exercise		
Having a chronic illness		
Other		

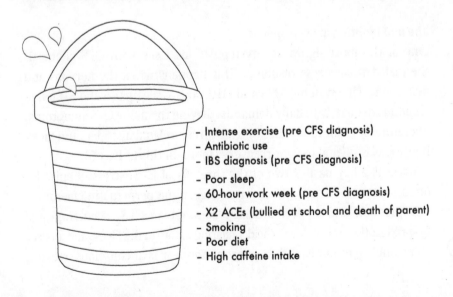

- Intense exercise (pre CFS diagnosis)
- Antibiotic use
- IBS diagnosis (pre CFS diagnosis)

- Poor sleep
- 60-hour work week (pre CFS diagnosis)

- X2 ACEs (bullied at school and death of parent)
- Smoking
- Poor diet
- High caffeine intake

The functional impact of chronic stress

One of the reasons why chronic stress poses such a threat to our health, especially if we have CFS, is that it disrupts the body's physiology. Here are some of the ways in which it contributes to dysregulation:

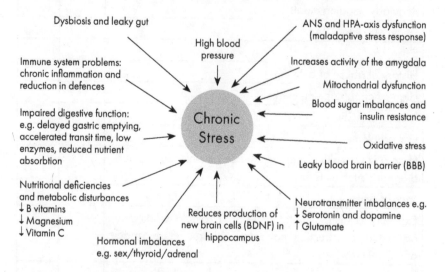

Dysbiosis and leaky gut

High blood pressure

ANS and HPA-axis dysfunction (maladaptive stress response)

Immune system problems: chronic inflammation and reduction in defences

Increases activity of the amygdala

Mitochondrial dysfunction

Impaired digestive function: e.g. delayed gastric emptying, accelerated transit time, low enzymes, reduced nutrient absorbtion

Blood sugar imbalances and insulin resistance

Oxidative stress

Chronic Stress

Leaky blood brain barrier (BBB)

Nutritional deficiencies and metabolic disturbances
↓ B vitamins
↓ Magnesium
↓ Vitamin C

Neurotransmitter imbalances e.g.
↓ Serotonin and dopamine
↑ Glutamate

Reduces production of new brain cells (BDNF) in hippocampus

Hormonal imbalances e.g. sex/thyroid/adrenal

Chronic stress leaves a dangerous cocktail of chemicals surging through the body, which wreaks havoc on our day-to-day functioning, causing wear and tear on our systems. As you can see, this feeds into the various other chronic stressors (deficiencies and toxicities) seen in the illness on p. 79. Therefore, stress (and trauma) are hugely important pieces of the jigsaw.

The maladaptive stress response

One of the most significant dysregulations I see with CFS clients is the maladaptive stress response. This happens when the nervous and neuroendocrine system (ANS and HPA-axis – see pp. 46 and 51) fail to respond adequately to daily demands, driving the many CFS symptoms. Therefore, it is fair to say that CFS is a stress-related disorder, and tackling stress is pivotal in your recovery (more on this in Part 3).

Stress is a key part of two of the three Ps of CFS: stressful episodes often precede CFS, and can occur as trigger and perpetuating factors.

Depression and anxiety are very common in CFS, occurring as a by-product (low mood due to the debilitating nature of the illness and anxiety about one's symptoms). Often, these can appear as unconscious stresses.

Free radicals and oxidative stress

Oxidative stress refers to a disturbance in the balance between the production of reactive oxygen species (known as free radicals) and anti-oxidant defences, constituting another chronic stressor in CFS.

Free radicals are unstable molecules that are missing an electron from their outer shell. For them to become stable again, they go on a scavenger hunt to steal from other molecules, which, in turn, do the same to others, causing a cascade of cellular damage.

Antioxidants are substances that inhibit or slow the process of oxidation and work to protect our cellular health from free radicals. They can be found in certain foods, such as fruits and vegetables, and are also produced within the body.

When free radicals overwhelm our antioxidant defence systems, it is known as oxidative stress. Free radicals can be produced in the body (for example, in the mitochondria). However, certain lifestyle factors can also accelerate their production, such as:

- exposure to toxic chemicals, pesticides and air pollution
- smoking
- alcohol
- poor diet and nutritional deficiencies
- exercise (**note:** while physical activity increases free radicals in the short term, some studies link it to increased antioxidant production in the long term[32])
- UV radiation
- obesity
- psychological stress
- medication and drugs
- infections and inflammation.

Examples of antioxidants include:
- vitamins A, C and E
- carotenoids (such as beta-carotene, lycopene, lutein, zeaxanthin)
- polyphenols
- selenium

- zinc
- coenzyme Q10 (CoQ10)
- carnitine
- glutathione (produced by the body)
- superoxide dismutase (produced by the body)
- alpha lipoic acid (produced by the body).

Oxidative stress has been shown to damage DNA and contribute to cellular malfunctioning, including impairment of the mitochondria and driving chronic inflammation. Improving your antioxidant defence systems is therefore key to CFS recovery to protect the cells from injury (see p. 241).

Nutritional deficiency

There isn't a lot of published evidence on nutritional deficiency in CFS; however, some research links the illness with deficiencies of the following nutrients:

- B vitamins [33,34]
- Magnesium [35]
- Carnitine [36]
- CoQ10 [37]
- Glutathione [38]
- Omega-3 fatty acids (EPA and DHA) [39]

As well as the above, I often see deficiencies of vitamin D, iron, zinc and iodine in my clinical practice.

Let's not also forget that chronic stress switches off our ability to absorb nutrients from our diets (likely because it lowers stomach acid and digestive-enzyme levels). Perhaps the saying 'you are what you eat' should really be 'you are what you absorb'.

Nutritional deficiencies are another stress load on our functional body systems, but one that can easily be rectified. Blood and urine tests can examine how much of a certain nutrient you have available to you or may require; for more on this, as well as information on nutrition and supplementation, see Part 3 (pp. 118–120 and 177–179).

Anaemia and fatigue

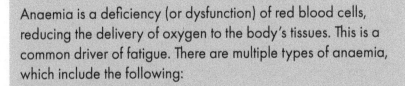

Anaemia is a deficiency (or dysfunction) of red blood cells, reducing the delivery of oxygen to the body's tissues. This is a common driver of fatigue. There are multiple types of anaemia, which include the following:

- **Iron-deficiency anaemia** When there isn't enough iron in the body, it cannot produce enough haemoglobin (a substance in red blood cells that enables them to carry oxygen around the tissues). See p. 168 for more information on iron deficiency and p. 114 for the best ways to test for it.

- **Anaemia resulting from other nutrient deficiencies, such as vitamin B 12 or folate** These can also impact the body's ability to produce fully functioning red blood cells, causing them to become abnormally large, which is why they are known as megaloblastic anaemias.

- **Pernicious anaemia** This is a specific type of vitamin-B 12-deficiency anaemia, caused by an autoimmune attack on cells in the stomach. The stomach produces a protein that is important for absorbing vitamin B 12 (known as intrinsic factor). When the body's immune system attacks these stomach cells, vitamin B 12 cannot be absorbed from the diet and, as a result, we develop a deficiency (in this way, pernicious anaemia is a form of megaloblastic anaemia).

Why some people get CFS and others do not

Many CFS patients ask me what makes some of us more susceptible to this illness than others.

We have established a genetic predisposition, but we can gain further insight from two other schools of thought, namely the 'germ' and 'terrain' theories of disease:

- **Germ theory** According to nineteenth-century French microbiologist Louis Pasteur, germ theory is the idea that microorganisms, such as viruses and bacteria, are what we need to worry about when dealing with illness.

- **Terrain theory**, argued by Antoine Béchamp, another nineteenth-century French scientist, posits that if the body is healthy and well balanced, it will deal with germs (which are a natural part of life), making us less susceptible to disease.

Luckily, we can influence our terrain by supporting the functioning of our body systems (such as the immune system, nervous system and microbiome) – cleaning up the body's environment to make the terrain healthier and ward off illness and microbe infiltration, so that it can appropriately deal with infections. Granted, it is also important to work on any chronic infections that are hindering health, which means that a combination of both the germ and terrain theories is needed when dealing with CFS.

We will further explore the importance of supporting the terrain and dealing with any infections in Part 3.

We have now covered some of the major drivers of CFS. However, as you have seen, it is multifaceted and involves a complex interplay between predisposition, trigger factors and chronic stressors (deficiencies and toxicities), which further drive physiological dysregulation, all of which add to your load.

Key takeaways

- Fatigue and the symptoms of CFS are an alarm system communicating that something is not quite right within the body and needs addressing.

- CFS can be viewed as a chronic physiological response to a storm of threats, such as a trigger infection, surgery, vaccination or trauma, compounded by a multitude of ongoing stressors.

- These chronic stressors can be grouped into 'deficiencies' and 'toxicities' (which include stress itself). In combination, these perpetuate symptoms of illness by causing poor cellular and physiological health. They also feed into one another, to form the complexity of CFS (for example, toxins, infections and nutritional deficiencies can impair mitochondrial function).

I understand that this has been a dense section, but I hope it has provided you with a better understanding of your condition and validation of your symptoms. And well done for getting through it!

Often, CFS involves a genetic predisposition combined with a culmination of stressors that lead the body to a tipping point (this might be an infection, vaccination, trauma, surgery or toxic chemical exposure). It is at this tipping point that the system crashes and struggles to restore balance, falling into a vicious cycle of endless symptoms perpetuated by chronic stressors (see figure on the next page).

As you can see, a culmination of stressors might have built up prior to your illness, until the tipping point, when your health starts to spiral into decline and CFS ensues. Sure, we all have stressors in our life; but, if there is a predisposition to CFS, then we are likely to fall unwell when we reach the final straw.

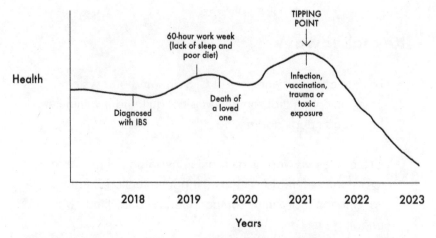

Before moving on to Part 3, you might find it helpful to create a time-line to help you make sense of how you got to where you are now. This might include:

- what your life was like before you became unwell
- triggers for your illness and what was happening in your life at the time you became unwell
- what happened after you became ill
- where you are now.

You could also include in your timeline where you want to be in the future.

We have so far covered an explanatory model for CFS that includes several factors: chronic infection, autoimmunity and immune disturbances, inflammation, mitochondrial problems, dysbiosis and imbalances in the neuroendocrine and autonomic nervous systems. These are all avenues that can be explored and investigated with your healthcare practitioner to help them establish which tests to consider, based on your presenting symptoms and concerns. (We look at testing in detail on pp. 112–123.)

I am sure that by now what you really want to know is what you can do to improve your health. Well, coming up very shortly in Part 3 are all the ways in which you can identify and address the various components of your system load to set you on the road to recovery and good health.

PART 3

The Road to Recovery

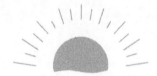

Now we get to the good part – the 'so-what-the-heck-do-I-do-next?' section.

In this part of the book, I am going to provide you with the tools and advice to get your body ticking over nicely and functioning in a much more helpful way.

This final section contains advice on handling the various aspects of daily life that are known to affect both energy and cognition. I know that fatigue is something that can really affect your concentration, so the advice here is designed to be easily digested and simple to put into practice yourself at home.

This information is supported by input from real-life clients who have attended my clinic and employed the various strategies within their own lives for recovery from CFS.

CHAPTER 9

First Steps

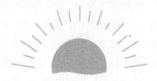

Believe you can and you're halfway there.
Theodore Roosevelt, twenty-sixth US President

Before we kick off with all the tips and advice, let's first explore what recovery looks like in real terms.

'Where do I even begin?'

These are often the wilderness times when you don't really get what the heck is going on, and you're not sure where – or how – to start your recovery journey. Not surprising, then, that I am frequently asked, 'Where do I even begin?'

We've all been there, and those initial stages of the illness are a confusing place to be. Hopefully, Part 2 has dispelled some of the anxiety (and the fog) around what is happening to your body in CFS; and applying the view that what you are experiencing is a form of dysregulation should have diffused some of the accompanying over-whelm, helping you to realise that steps can be taken to restore balance in your health and life.

Getting a diagnosis

Firstly, if you suspect that you have CFS and are experiencing the various symptoms listed on p. 28, along with identifying a possible trigger episode (such as an infection, surgery or immunisation), it is important to visit your GP for them to investigate further.

One of the difficulties we face is that medical training in CFS (and, of course, for long COVID, too) is still falling short. Some doctors might attribute your symptoms to a 'self-limiting condition', which is a term used to describe an illness that resolves itself naturally, without any medical treatment. Others may still be adopting a psychological approach to the illness and blaming your fatigue (and other symptoms) on depression or mental-health problems. And there are still some doctors who simply do not 'believe in' CFS – I would, of course, avoid them like the plague!

Fortunately, however, the tide is turning, and many doctors are now much more clued into CFS than ever before (we have the COVID pandemic to thank for this). Regardless, you should ensure that you consult a doctor who is open-minded and supportive, and who fully acknowledges CFS and its *physical basis* as a condition. (You might like to show them this book and Part 2 in particular!)

If your GP does not fit the bill, you are perfectly within your rights to keep asking for a second or third opinion, until you are satisfied. You could either ask the receptionist at your current practice if any of the doctors there have experience of working with patients with CFS (or other complex chronic illnesses) or, if necessary, ask for a referral to another local surgery or practice.

If your memory and concentration aren't particularly good when you attend appointments, then take a partner or friend or relative with you who may be able to help discuss your health on your behalf.

A doctor should take a good clinical history, listen to you carefully and ask the right types of questions as you provide your medical information. Questions should include things like the following:

- How long have your symptoms been going on for?
- How are your symptoms affecting your ability to undertake daily

tasks and activities, compared with previously?

- Are there any events or illnesses (such as catching an infection) that you associate with the onset of your symptoms?

They might also perform some physical examinations, as well as routine blood and urine tests.

As I mentioned earlier, since there is no medical test to diagnose CFS, investigations will be undertaken to rule out any other potential causes of your symptoms. Only when nothing else has been identified will a doctor diagnose you with CFS.

Note: some people never receive a formal diagnosis of CFS (like myself), but this doesn't necessarily mean that you do not have it. And since there isn't an awful lot that the medical profession can offer, a diagnosis of CFS may not really seem to be worth much. However, it can be seen as important from a medical standpoint to have alternative diagnoses ruled out and to gain some understanding about your health.

Explaining CFS to friends and family

Once you have received a CFS diagnosis – or at the very least ruled out all other possibilities – the next step is to share this information with your friends and family, your boss and work colleagues – a tricky task when the illness itself is so misunderstood within society and modern medicine.

Explain that you are currently unwell with CFS, a fluctuating illness that dysregulates your body systems (including the nervous, neuro-endocrine and immune systems), and how this means that some of the activities you used to do may be a little bit more challenging, and that you must make decisions regarding your daily activity and lifestyle habits to support your health.

How much depth you go into will depend largely on who you are speaking to, which is why it is important to gauge how receptive somebody is to your news and to judge the information you impart accordingly. I say this because I have come across more than my fair share of naysayers who have doubted the condition and its impact on my life. (The misconception that all CFS sufferers are bed or wheel-chair-bound, and that you have to look unwell to have CFS, is still rife.) And as sad as it is, there is no point wasting your precious energy (which is already severely limited) on people who are closed-minded.

Seek instead the comfort of supportive people. Hopefully, in the future society will gain a greater understanding of CFS, and the stigma will reduce (we are already starting to see signs of this since the pandemic), but, in the meantime, stick with those who will be empathetic to your situation and share your experiences with those you can trust.

It's not your fault!

Many sufferers blame themselves for their situation, and while it's true that this illness can impact your self-esteem (probably because you aren't able to function like you used to), please remember that you are not lazy, despite the fact that you (or even other people) might feel that this is the case.

In fact, CFS sufferers are among the strongest group of people I have ever met, given that they often conceal their suffering and try to 'push through' the pain and symptoms. Which is not to say that pushing your-self is a good thing (we will talk more about this later), but it certainly demonstrates a strength of character.

The Spoon Theory

The Spoon Theory story was written by lupus sufferer Christine Miserandino as a metaphor for what it is like to live with chronic illness. Using spoons as a unit of energy, it proposes the idea that people with chronic disease only get a handful of spoons each day and have to decide how to use these limited reserves.

This idea became so popular that many hashtags on social media popped up as a result, with chronic illness sufferers identifying as a '#spoonie'.

The Spoon Theory may be useful to people who are trying to understand more of what you are dealing with following your diagnosis and who are open to learning about CFS. Simply search 'the spoon theory' online for more information.

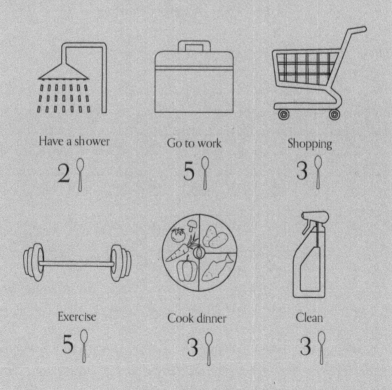

Have a shower
2

Go to work
5

Shopping
3

Exercise
5

Cook dinner
3

Clean
3

CHAPTER 10

Is Recovery Possible?

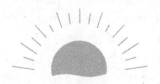

If you change the way you look at things,
the things you look at change.
Wayne Dyer, American author

It may seem tough to keep a positive outlook when suffering with CFS, but I believe that *it is possible to recover your health.*

Now some of you may feel a twinge of cynicism here. You might be thinking, It's too good to be true – I've tried absolutely everything, and I still haven't recovered; maybe Lauren is just one of the lucky ones . . .

Well, I'm with you on this and I have shared your scepticism along the way. In fact, these are the same thoughts that I had throughout my years of ill health and my incessant repetition of the question: is recovery from CFS even possible?

And there's another layer of uncertainty on top of this, which many of my clients express, namely, 'Will I ever be *fully* recovered, or will I only ever be "managing" my illness?'

These are valid questions, and it is natural to want to understand what your future looks like, and whether you will always be living under the cloud of chronic illness or if you will be free from its clutches.

One of the most important things to say here is that belief is a fundamental force in influencing your recovery from CFS. This might sound completely woo-woo but hear me out.

This illness and its very nature are almost the opposite of what you know – and so is the route out of it. I will explain to you exactly why belief (or indeed, suspending your *dis*belief) is a pivotal first step in the recovery journey as we move through this section.

It's important to remember that your healthcare professionals' opinions will have been shaped by their own experiences of the illness and not necessarily by any statistical data, per se. With this in mind, walk yourself back to your first prognosis. Who was the healthcare professional? What did they say to you? Were they optimistic or pessimistic? Consider the words used around your diagnosis.

The chances are that this opinion may have influenced your outlook during your illness and that your *beliefs* on recovery will be shaped by it. So many people think they are doomed because they hear negative stories from their doctors about the illness being 'incurable' and 'lifelong'.

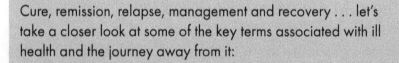

The language of recovery

Cure, remission, relapse, management and recovery . . . let's take a closer look at some of the key terms associated with ill health and the journey away from it:

- **Cure:** a substance (for example, a medical drug) or procedure that ends a medical condition
- **Remission:** a temporary end to (or lessening in severity of) a disease
- **Relapse:** a deterioration in health after a period of improvement; can also be defined as a return to ill health
- **Management:** maintaining control over, coping, or withstanding something
- **Recovery:** a process through which there is an improvement in health and wellbeing; a return to any former and/or better state or condition

The word 'cure' is not applicable to CFS. While remission is perhaps somewhat more appropriate, it implies only a 'temporary' end to illness, which has negative connotations (plus, it's not necessarily accurate, as many CFS patients do experience complete recovery). Similarly, the words 'relapse' and 'management' are also quite negative, while management implies that there is an illness still there to be suppressed, controlled or withstood.

We must not place ourselves in this box of negative thinking when considering the possibility of achieving better health. Which is where 'recovery' comes in.

A recovery is a process of transformation with an upward trajectory from ill health towards better health. As such, this is one of the most useful ways to look at this illness.

Who said recovery isn't possible?

Some people think that they will only ever be 'managing' their condition and therefore they are buying into a static version of their health. But if you think of your health as fluid and *believe* that recovery is possible, it becomes far easier to move forwards – after all, beliefs are simply opinions, yet we so often treat them as facts.

A useful message I like to tell my clients is that:

> *If something is not impossible, then, all of a sudden*
> (by some margin), *it becomes possible.*

On the positive side, recovery can be full (i.e. complete) or partial. Sometimes we get so hung up on overanalysing our symptoms and aiming to be 100-per-cent symptom-free that we fail to see the incredible progress we have made so far. So instead of thinking, I'm not there yet, think: Look how far I have come. A partial recovery is never static

– it means you are on that upward trajectory towards a better level of physical functioning; and it also gives you some psychological wiggle room to know that you aren't staying in that place for ever, and that full recovery in the future is also a real possibility.

The stages of recovery

There are three notable stages of recovery from CFS:

- **The crash stage** This is when the illness first hits and you are feeling an overwhelming sense of fatigue. In this stage, you are likely to be sleeping a lot and symptom severity will be at an all-time high.

- **The 'wired-and-tired' stage** Your body is starting to recoup some energy, which might seem like good news on the surface, but this energy is going straight towards your nervous system and contributing to high levels of stress and anxiety. So your body is still likely to be exhausted, and your mind is overactive – hence the wired-and-tired label.

- **The restoration stage** This is when you establish a stable baseline (where you feel healthy, and symptoms are much less apparent or even not present at all) and can start to reintegrate into normal life again. It can be a balancing act of trying not to overdo things to avoid crashing and a resurgence of symptoms, but it is a process of learning to trust your body a lot more and experimenting with new activities again (whether housework, socialising, work or exercise).

Sometimes, you will cycle back and forth between these three stages. For example, you might feel you are in stage 3, but then revert to stage 2 – and that's ok! It is all part of the process, so try to see it as a learning curve and not a setback.

We will explore how to best navigate these three stages in the lifestyle section on pp. 214–239.

How long will it take?

People often ask how long recovery takes, and it's a hard question to answer. The reality is that people recover in their own time and at their own pace. There is certainly no overnight fix and I generally tend to say that six to twelve months should be factored in as a bare minimum for solid improvements.

Having said that, the most important thing is to focus on the process and your progress, rather than on an end goal. The likelihood with this illness is that you won't just wake up one day and suddenly feel better. Patience is a pill we all need to swallow, but it's a gift that keeps on giving, and we learn so much along the way on this journey.

How do I get better?

First things first – there is no one single magic bullet or course of action that will get you well. In my own experience, and what I have found and experienced with clients, a combination of modes and methods work in tandem to move the needle in your wellbeing. A change in diet can offer dramatic benefits, for example, especially when combined with approaches like pacing activity levels and supporting the stress response.

The recovery rollercoaster: what recovery really looks like

I'm going to be very honest and pragmatic here (just as I am with my clients) and tell you that the journey to recovery from CFS is a tricky one. There are days when you just feel like giving up – when you want to throw in the towel and stop trying because, well, what's the point? Then there are days when you reach a huge milestone and you look back and think, Wow! I can't believe I have come this far.

The diagram below is a good representation of the often tortuous path from poor health to vibrant health.

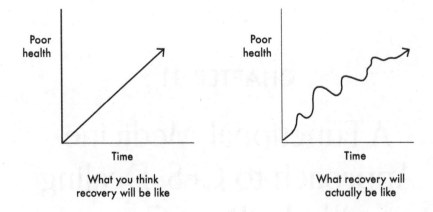

Poor health

Time

**What you think
recovery will be like**

Poor health

Time

**What recovery will
actually be like**

Recovery often seems like a wobbly rollercoaster ride of emotions and frequent setbacks. But if you take a closer look at the line on the diagram and the course that it is taking, you will see that, despite all the wobbles, you are generally moving forwards towards a stage of recovery. So whenever you are going through a low point, a crash or a setback, refer to this diagram and be reassured that even when it does not seem like it, you are always on course and moving in the right direction towards optimum health.

Work on practising acceptance. One of the greatest things you can do for yourself is to resist the resistance. Avoid fighting your symptoms, ride the waves and try to understand your triggers, so that you can move forwards.

CHAPTER 11

A Functional-Medicine Approach to CFS: Dealing with the Root Cause

We must all suffer from one of two pains: the pain of discipline or the pain of regret. The difference is that discipline weighs ounces, while regret weighs tons.
Jim Rohn, American entrepreneur

Functional medicine is an integrative model of healthcare that asks how and why illness occurs and aims to restore health by addressing the root cause. It is individualised and patient-centred with a physiology- and systems-based approach. Functional medicine is medicine by cause, not by symptom, and, as the diagram opposite shows, a diagnosis can be the result of more than just one factor. For example, CFS may be driven by infection, dysbiosis, mitochondrial problems and neuroendocrine imbalances.

My job is not to treat disease (I am not a doctor), but I work on the body's ecosystem – getting rid of the bad stuff, restoring the good and allowing the body's intelligent system to do the rest, finding its natural equilibrium.

The basis of functional-medicine practice is to view the patient as an individual, rather than focusing on the disease itself. It asks how the body is influenced by its environment, lifestyle and genetics, considering the triggers of poor health and lifestyle changes that can be made to combat health problems and promote wellness. That's why I look at the body as one whole, integrated system, while also assessing what is driving the illness and any lifestyle factors that may be involved in the perpetuation of symptoms.

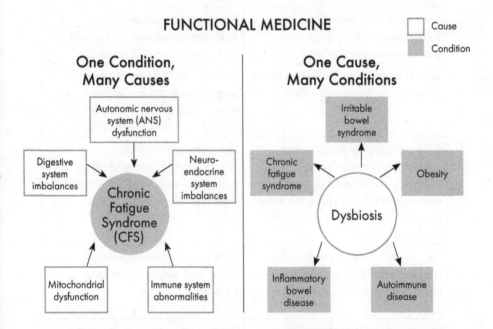

While reviewing biochemical system pathways and physiological processes, a functional-medicine practitioner would typically look at the following:

- Nutritional status
- Hormonal, immune, gut, cellular and genetic health
- Environmental and toxic burden
- Physical activity
- Sleep patterns
- Stress levels
- Emotional and mental state

This model also emphasises the importance of hearing somebody's story and calls for mindfulness of a patient's unique narrative. I personally know the value of having my story heard when a ten-minute GP appointment wouldn't quite cut it.

Functional medicine	Conventional medicine
Patient-centred with an understanding of what optimal health looks like	**Disease-centred** with a solid understanding of what poor health looks like
Each patient is **treated as an individual** with unique genetics, environments and lifestyles	**Treatments are often standardised** and not based on an individual's specific needs
Sees **the body as one whole system** that is interconnected	Looks at the body as **separate organ systems**. For example, you would typically consult a cardiologist for heart-related conditions
Uses principles of biology and physiology to **understand primary drivers of disease** and develops protocols to disable these drivers, often enabling symptoms to resolve themselves	Uses principles of biology and physiology to **form a diagnosis** and design treatments to alleviate symptoms of an illness
Focuses on the **root cause of a disease** and what underlying processes are involved in its aetiology	Beneficial for understanding the impacts on **separate organ systems** in disease
Focuses on the **triggers** of illness	Looks at the impacts of ill health (i.e., **symptom-focused**)
Considers what needs to be **improved upon** (e.g., nutrition, physical activity, sleep) and what should be ruled out (e.g. smoking, drugs)	Treats according to **protocol** and **guidelines**
Particularly beneficial for **chronic disease**	Beneficial for **acute disease and medical emergencies**
Considers **why** the illness is happening in the first place and looking at **how can we reverse this?**	Aims to firstly **diagnose the disease** and work out how to **alleviate symptoms and prevent progression**
Places heavy emphasis on lifestyle changes, while working alongside nutritional supplements and pharmaceutical medications, where appropriate	**Uses pharmaceutical medications** where appropriate, but often **overlooks lifestyle interventions** within common practice

Takes time and involves patient's active participation	Minimal time available for the patient's story to be heard
Uses scientific evidence base	Also uses scientific evidence base
Practised by doctors, as well as other healthcare professionals	Practised by doctors and other healthcare professionals

Now I'm not knocking traditional medicine by any means, and certainly, for anyone who has been in a car accident or had a heart attack, their local A&E is going to be their first port of call to save their life. However, when dealing with chronic disease, conventional Western medicine unfortunately does not have all the answers.

My clinical practice

Using a functional-medicine approach, my clinical practice focuses on personalisation when it comes to recovery from CFS. This is because no two CFS clients are alike, and it is probable that each has their own unique collection of chronic stressors driving their illness (along with possible co-morbidities that might occur on top of this – see p. 32). Therefore, there is no one standard protocol for everyone with CFS, and therapy is highly individualised.

I often liken health to an onion: as I work with my clients, it is like I am peeling back the layers to get to the bottom of what is going on. This forms the basis of our investigative work together, as we employ a variety of strategies to move the needle in their health.

I start by taking a thorough medical case history and assessing the main presenting symptoms and health concerns. We cover each of the body systems, going into more detail for those predominantly affected in CFS. I also ask you to provide a food diary, so that I can learn about your current diet.

As I always say, I can act as your satnav, but you are the one who must drive the car. Working with me requires a collaborative approach and your active engagement and commitment to the process are paramount, otherwise it just does not work. I am simply a guide to understanding your illness and a facilitator of the process and possibility of progress. But ultimately, your health is in your own hands, and you can hugely influence its course, through appropriate lifestyle and behavioural techniques.

CFS is an illness that requires an *active* rather than a passive approach to recovery. It's a process that requires time, patience and faith. Working on your health involves absolute commitment. Unfortunately, this often only occurs when the pain of where you are is greater than the pain of making changes, which tends to push this commitment forwards. It's a case of desperation fuelling inspiration. But eventually, you can really achieve wonders.

The key pillars of recovery

Before diving into the strategies that support improvements, I want to highlight the three key pillars of CFS recovery:

- Nutrition
- Lifestyle
- Mindset

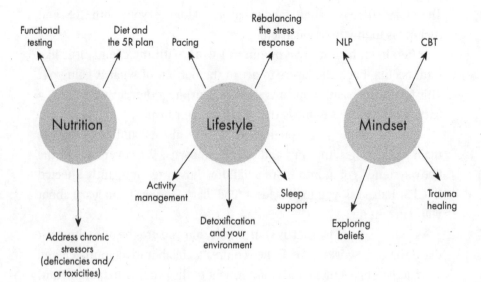

In CFS, it is hard to strike a balance between therapies that are 100 per cent evidence-based and those that are supported by some margin of evidence rooted in a solid scientific rationale. Granted, it does mean that you are taking more of a financial gamble (if the therapies in question cost money), but if there is value in learning something from an intervention, the possibility of a benefit for CFS symptoms and no risk of harm, then this should not be totally discounted.

The FM approach is an empowering tool for self-discovery, helping to peel back the layers of your health and provide strategies to optimise your level of physical functioning and recovery from CFS. Testing is a key factor underpinning the FM approach, and we will be exploring this in detail in the next chapter.

CHAPTER 12

Testing

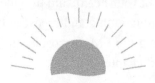

What the caterpillar calls the end of the world,
the master calls a butterfly.
Richard Bach, American author

In my clinical work-up, I will typically examine a client's case and there-after recommend some functional testing, that allows us to discover any imbalances and dysregulations that may lie at the heart of somebody's symptoms.

Functional testing can uncover unique health insights that can help to inform client protocols. Testing also opens a window for clients, so that they can understand the potential drivers of their symptoms, propelling them forwards in making solid lifestyle changes.

Unfortunately, functional testing is not available on the NHS and does, therefore, come at a client's own expense. However, there are some exceptions if you are fortunate enough to have private medical insurance, as some tests are covered under BUPA and AXA, for example (for more information on labs that do functional testing, see Resources, p. 308).

Finding the right solution to your chronic fatigue can be a long process that requires detective work to establish the root cause(s). And testing can be a great way to establish where to aim interventions and implement strategic and targeted lifestyle and nutritional change. My job, then, is to look at the individual in front of me and put my detective hat on, as I assess the clinical clues to their unique situation and panoply of CFS symptoms.

Ultimately, no one lab test will uncover all the dysfunctions in a CFS patient, so with functional testing it is about unpicking the mosaic of fatigue and creating a personalised action plan.

What is functional testing, and how does it differ from NHS testing?

A functional test, as its name suggests, examines how well the body is functioning. It will usually involve either a blood, saliva, breath, urine or stool sample, performed by private laboratories, which you can access through a healthcare provider, such as a nutritional therapist or naturo-path. Most samples can be taken at home, but on occasion a blood draw from a nurse or phlebotomist may be required.

In the NHS, testing uses markers that instantly pick up a disease or diagnosis, whereas functional testing typically examines dysfunction, using markers backed up by a large body of clinical data.

Functional testing also often assesses more markers than NHS tests – for example when testing thyroid function, the NHS typically looks at two markers, whereas functional testing measures eight, so providing more insight on how the thyroid is functioning. It also applies tighter reference ranges, allowing for earlier detection of problems, such as an underactive thyroid gland, helping to stop it in its tracks and prevent it from progressing into a diagnosis of hypothyroidism in the future.

In this way, functional tests can provide insights on dysfunction versus absolute disease, assessing physiology in dynamic and exciting new ways.

Importantly, functional testing helps us to answer the question 'Why?' Why is a symptom occurring? Is there an underlying thyroid problem that has not been properly identified? Are the adrenals strained and not producing adequate levels of cortisol? Or is the gut out of balance – are there any underlying infections, nutritional deficiencies or toxic over-loads that may be impairing the mitochondria and driving the boatload of chronic stressors within the body? This is where the saying 'Test, don't guess' comes in useful.

It is a means of self-discovery for many of my clients, allowing them, with me, to dig deeper and uncover the biochemical imbalances that explain their symptoms. And while these tests are by no means diagnostic, they do provide a key piece of the puzzle towards achieving better overall health.

Initial tests to request from your GP

I generally ask that my clients request some standard tests, free of charge, from their GP, including the following:

- Full blood count
- Full iron panel (this includes serum ferritin, total/serum iron, transferrin/total iron binding capacity, and transferrin saturation)
- Vitamin D (25(OH)D), folate and vitamin B12 (if you can, see if you can also test for active B12, known as holotranscobalamin, which is the type that your body is most able to use)
- Blood glucose (HbA1C and fasting blood glucose)
- Thyroid function (TSH and FT4)
- Uric acid
- Liver function
- Lipid profile
- ESR and C-reactive protein
- Electrolytes
- Blood pressure

Other tests that may be useful from your doctor include the following:

- Homocysteine (high levels can be a further indicator of low B vitamin status – B6, B9, B12, for example)

- Infectious pathogens (such as EBV, mycoplasma, cytomegalovirus, Borrelia)
- Anti-nuclear antibodies (ANA) (to see if there is autoimmune activity)
- Intrinsic factor antibodies (to see if there is pernicious anaemia)
- Serum tryptase (helpful if there is suspected mast cell activation syndrome, MCAS)
- Diamine oxidase (DAO) (to assess for histamine intolerance)
- Tilt-table test or NASA lean test (to assess for orthostatic intolerance)

I would also recommend that you ensure that your doctor screens you for other conditions that may be causing your symptoms, such as coeliac disease, inflammatory bowel disease or multiple sclerosis.

It can sometimes be a challenge getting doctors to perform a battery of tests, but I'd advise that you state your case in terms of your need to rule out potential causes of your symptoms with a view to identifying the most appropriate next steps to take. (These tests are just a starting point, and won't provide the same level of detail as functional testing.)

What functional tests are available?

Testing is carried out on an individualised basis, depending on the main presenting symptoms and case history. There are many functional tests available, but the following are most useful in helping to identify the chronic stressors we so often see in CFS:

- Adrenal testing
- Microbiome analysis
- Thyroid dysfunction

- Chronic-infection testing (including chronic Lyme disease)
- Organic-acids testing
- Nutritional (vitamin and mineral) testing
- Genetic testing
- Toxicity testing

Now let's dive into what these tests are and what they involve in more detail.

Adrenal testing

Adrenal gland imbalance (also known as HPA axis dysfunction) happens when real or perceived stress becomes too much for the body to handle. As we saw on p. 52, stress hormones such as cortisol can be either too high or too low – however, the former can lead to the latter, which is why (due to the body being stuck in fight-or-flight mode) it is common to see adrenal insufficiency in CFS.

Salivary sampling is one of the most accurate ways of assessing steroid hormone levels because it measures free cortisol (the active form of cortisol) and is a more accurate representation of how the hormone is used within the body. A functional adrenal assessment can see whether you have elevated levels of cortisol and DHEA (a hormone produced by the adrenal glands, which counterbalances the destructive effects caused by long periods of high cortisol) or, indeed, whether the levels of these hormones have become insufficient to keep up with the body's daily demands.

If you are someone with a history of chronic stress in your life, compounded by blood-sugar imbalances, fatigue or sleeping difficulties, then a salivary adrenal test might also be useful in determining how out of balance these glands really are.

While long-term stress is the major driver of adrenal insufficiency, other causes can include a poor diet, lack of sleep, emotional trauma, too much exercise and toxic exposure, which can all tax your adrenals.

Microbiome analysis

A microbiome test is a stool test that examines gastrointestinal function in detail. It can assess:

- levels of digestive enzymes
- dysbiosis (including the detection of SIBO – see p. 73; however, the gold standard for this is always a breath test)
- inflammation
- infections (pathogenic bacteria, Candida, H. pylori, parasites)
- metabolite imbalance (i.e. short-chain fatty acids).

Stool testing is one of the tests I tend to use the most in clinic because the gut opens a window on to the health of the entire body, including the nervous and immune systems. Therefore, identifying any imbalances in this area is critical when it comes to CFS, particularly for somebody who has myriad digestive issues (such as IBS) as part of their clinical picture.

Thyroid dysfunction

I always advise a standard GP thyroid test for those struggling with CFS, but it is certainly worthwhile considering a functional thyroid assessment, too. This is especially relevant if you have a goitre (a lump in the front of the neck caused by swelling of the thyroid gland) or a family history of autoimmune disease.

However, I also recommend full functional thyroid blood tests because standard thyroid testing does not provide a complete picture of how the gland is performing, since most NHS doctors will only test for TSH and T4 levels.

A functional thyroid assessment may therefore be useful in helping CFS patients understand where their thyroid hormone levels sit, which can better explain or rule out thyroid dysfunction. As mentioned earlier, they use advanced markers and tighter reference ranges which can help to identify more thyroid problems and spot them earlier on. I would advise regular check-ups on your thyroid gland, particularly if you are female and over the age of fifty, as your risk of hypothyroidism increases.

Chronic-infection testing

Testing for infection is available on the NHS, but it is also possible to perform some functional tests that can examine whether there are any common pathogens associated with CFS at play, including the following:

- Borrelia burgdorferi (the bacteria that causes Lyme disease)
- Anaplasma
- Chlamydia pneumoniae (can cause pneumonia)
- Yersinia
- Epstein–Barr virus (EBV – causes infectious mononucleosis, aka mono or glandular fever)
- Cytomegalovirus
- Coxsackievirus (can cause hand, foot and mouth disease)
- Babesia
- Bartonella
- Mycoplasma (can, in some cases, cause pneumonia – often known as 'walking pneumonia' because it is usually mild and doesn't require hospitalisation)
- Varicella-zoster virus (causes chickenpox/shingles)
- Ehrlichia

NHS tests commonly measure IgG and IgM antibodies when it comes to identifying infectious pathogens. IgG antibodies are generally taken to be a sign of a past infection and can stay elevated in the blood for many years, while IgM antibodies only remain for a few weeks following an infection, after which they start to disappear (even if the infection has not gone). So these may not be a good indicator of whether an active infection is at work.

Functional tests examine specific white blood cells, which can signal the presence of active infection.

Organic-acids testing

Organic acids (OAs) are carbon-containing compounds that are breakdown products of amino acids, carbs and fats, as well as neurotransmitters and even intestinal bacteria.

The analysis of OAs with a urine test can inform us about the body's ability to generate energy (from the mitochondria) and detoxify harmful environmental toxins, as well as provide key insights into vitamin and mineral requirements, oxidative stress, neurotransmitters and the health of the gastrointestinal (GI) tract (microbiome).

OA testing vs nutrient screening

It is easy to mistake OA tests for an indication of overall nutritional status, but the biochemical markers measured in an OA test simply give an indication of somebody's increased need for a particular nutrient, even if there is no clinical deficiency.

However, it is possible to screen for nutritional status through blood testing, which provides an indication of nutrient levels within the body. Nutrient tests are a little bit like going into the bank and checking your balance, whereas OA tests are like bank statements that show you where you've spent your money, or if there have been any problems paying the bills. OA tests examine metabolic pathways, which can indicate what nutrients there may be an increased demand for to support metabolic functions (such as energy production in the mitochondria), whereas standard nutrient tests can reveal what vitamins and minerals you have available to you already (more on this below).

Nutritional (vitamin and mineral) testing

It can be very useful to assess nutrient levels in CFS, particularly because many sufferers tend to have deficiencies in some of the key vitamins and minerals required for energy production, including the following:

- Magnesium
- B vitamins – B1, B2, B3, B5, B6, B7, B9 (folate) and B12
- Iron
- Iodine
- Selenium
- Vitamin C
- Vitamin D
- Zinc
- CoQ10

- Carnitine
- Alpha lipoic acid (ALA)
- Glutathione
- Nicotinamide adenine dinucleotide (NAD+)

I run comprehensive nutrient tests to gain a picture of patients' nutritional status. While it is possible to have the healthiest and most nutritious diet on the surface, if you are not appropriately absorbing your nutrients you are much more prone to deficiencies (we discuss how to tackle absorption problems on pp. 171–172).

Genetic testing

Genetic testing has become a popular tool for exploring an individual's health in greater detail. It usually involves a mouth swab to collect DNA to identify genetic variants called SNPs (single nucleotide polymorphisms, pronounced 'snips'). Most chronic diseases occur via an interplay between gene variants and epigenetic factors.

Epigenetics is a growing area of scientific interest that studies external factors that affect the way in which our genes work – because while our genetic blueprints are predetermined from birth, environment and lifestyle pull the trigger on how these genes are expressed. Therefore epigenetics (which literally means 'on top of' genetics) refers to the external factors that can turn genes 'on' or 'off'.

But how is epigenetics relevant to CFS? Well, one of the things it looks at is a process called methylation – a chemical reaction in the body in which a small molecule (known as a methyl group) is added to DNA, proteins or other molecules, potentially affecting the way in which some molecules act in the body (as well as having the ability to switch genes off or silence them). Methylation plays a major role in most of the body's cellular metabolic functions, occurring billions of times every single second. Some of the jobs it has a helping hand in include:

- switching genes off
- detoxifying chemicals and toxins from the body
- building neurotransmitters
- breaking down hormones and supporting hormonal balance

- building immune cells
- energy production
- histamine metabolism
- supporting liver and nervous-system health
- fat burning.

If the body is under-methylating, several important molecules cannot be efficiently produced to support energy production, including:

- glutathione
- CoQ10
- melatonin
- serotonin
- nitric oxide
- epinephrine (adrenaline)
- norepinephrine (noradrenaline)
- carnitine
- cysteine.

Learning whether or not you are a good methylator is important because it can provide clues as to how to bypass bottlenecks and weaknesses in certain biochemical pathways that specifically affect energy production and physiological health. Vitamins (in particular B2, B6, B9 and B12 – see p. 162), minerals and amino acids from the diet are needed to keep the methylation process running smoothly.

In the context of CFS, genetic testing can be helpful in determining the presence of genetic variants that may contribute to the overall picture of fatigue.

Genetic testing can also tell us how well our bodies process and eliminate toxins, metabolise histamine and process and absorb vitamin B12, as well as our propensity to handle and metabolise certain foods, such as dairy (lactose), gluten (coeliac-disease risk) and caffeine. These are all relevant to our understanding of CFS on an individualised level.

Ⓘ

Toxicity testing

Toxicity testing can be useful if CFS onset is associated with environmental exposures or if there is a suspected burden of toxic stress in somebody who has been in high-risk situations, such as:

- agriculture and farming (exposure to organophosphate pesticides)
- living or working in a damp, mouldy environment with poor ventilation (exposure to mould)
- someone with a history of amalgam fillings (exposure to mercury)
- consuming lots of high-mercury fish (including swordfish, tuna, king mackerel)
- working as a pilot or cabin crew or frequent flying for other reasons (exposure to organophosphates in engine oils)
- outdoor and indoor pollution (traffic and exhaust fumes, cosmetics, household chemicals, sprays and cleaning agents, aluminium deodorants, flame-retardant mattresses, aluminium or Teflon pans).

We are all regularly exposed to toxins so, even if you do not think you have been in an obviously high-risk situation that predisposes you to toxicity, it is certainly a factor worth exploring, particularly if there is multiple chemical sensitivity (MCS) present.

Most toxicity tests are taken via blood or urine and can help to see what is impeding the smooth running of someone's liver, biochemical pathways and physiological functioning, triggering fatigue-related issues.

Functional testing and health anxiety

Speaking from my own experience, I held so much anxiety around the results of functional tests that it clouded my judgement on my wellbeing and CFS recovery.

At a certain point in the process, it is more important to go by how your body intrinsically *feels*, rather than the results of a functional test. For example, if a test shows that you have adrenal insufficiency, but your energy levels are starting to improve, focus on that, rather than on attaining the 'perfect' test result. This is especially important for adrenal health, because sometimes we can try too hard to get better, placing unwanted strain on the nervous system.

Another example is chronic infections. I've seen many clients get hung up on a positive test result, but it is important to remember that some infections do stay with us for life. Herpes is one such infection. This does not mean that everyone who harbours the herpes virus is going to present with symptoms (such as cold sores). In fact, some will never even know that they have it, which means that we can co-exist with certain microbes and be healthy.

Certainly, in CFS it is important to address and pay consideration to any pathogens that may be lurking because they *may* be contributing to the boatload of symptoms experienced. It may also be a question of pathogenic load and how the immune system behaves in response, which can be influenced and improved through dietary and lifestyle measures.

Functional testing has a valid place in the puzzle that is CFS but try not to dwell on results or place your recovery hopes on this alone. Testing is a guideline for your current health status – a roadmap – but nothing can replace your personal understanding and intuition as to how your body feels and its inherent needs.

CHAPTER 13

Nutrition I – Your Diet and the 5R Plan

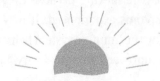

Your diet is like a bank account.
Good food choices are good investments.
Bethenny Frankel, American businesswoman
and TV personality

Did you know that the food you eat can influence your energy levels, gene expression, hormones, brain chemistry, mood, immunity, digestive wellbeing and so much more? So given the role of the various system dysregulations in CFS, it makes sense that food plays a starring role in getting people back to vibrant health.

The following key can be used when consulting lists of foods throughout this chapter; if you have FODMAP, histamine or sulphur intolerances (pp. 127–128), it will help with making decisions as to which foods to include versus which to go easy on.

Key: **F** = high FODMAP (see p. 126); **H** = high histamine; **S** = high sulphur

What diet is suitable for CFS recovery?

There is no one-size-fits-all diet when it comes to CFS. However, understanding the importance of nutrition, even on a cellular and biochemical level, is crucial with this illness. Which is why nutritional changes are key to my work in clinic – because, after all, we are dealing with a dysregulated physiological system.

I love helping my clients to find a way of eating that supports their health and ensures that they are receiving adequate levels of nutrients to ward off fatigue and any other symptoms that they may be experiencing.

The importance of bio-individuality

Vegetarian . . . Paleo . . . Sugar-free . . . Yeast-free . . . Gluten-free . . . Dairy-free . . . You name it, I've probably tried it!

I have had my own encounters with various healing diets over the years, and, after practising in clinic for some years now and seeing numerous clients on their own CFS journeys, I am a firm believer in the concept of bio-individuality.

Bio-individuality means that each person is biochemically unique, with highly individualised nutritional requirements, which can be deciphered from internal factors (such as genetics, hormones, immune tolerance, metabolism, nutritional status and gut health), as well as external ones (such as stress levels and lifestyle patterns).

That said, I like to marry the concept of bio-individuality with some basic nutritional common sense when it comes to rooted-in-science dietary principles that will suit the majority of CFS sufferers out there. This is because, despite each CFS patient being unique, I do also see common patterns among clients.

Food intolerance and food sensitivity in CFS

Although we have acknowledged that there may not be sufficient data to say, 'Follow X diet and you will get better from CFS', what *is* clear is that food sensitivities and intolerances are rife in many CFS patients. And this proves the case for using elimination diets as a recovery tool.

The most common food intolerances and sensitivities include gluten, dairy (to lactose, casein or whey), fructose, eggs, wheat, yeast, FODMAPs (fermentable short-chain carbohydrates found naturally in various foods), histamine, caffeine, alcohol, sulphur, salicylates, night-shades (due to the high alkaloid content) and sulphites.

There is often a lot of confusion between the terms 'food intolerance', 'food sensitivity' and 'food allergy', so for clarity's sake, let's establish the difference between the three:

What is a food allergy?

In an allergic reaction, the body mistakes a particular food for a threat, causing mild to severe symptoms (in some cases, these can be life-threatening). Food allergies trigger an almost immediate onset of symptoms after the offending food has been ingested – usually from a few minutes to two hours after eating the food – in the form of tingling or itching in the mouth, swelling of the face, mouth and tongue (known as angioedema), difficulty swallowing, skin rashes and anaphylaxis (which causes severe breathing difficulties). Some symptoms, particularly anaphylaxis, can be life-threatening, and urgent medical attention is required if you suspect that someone is having an allergic reaction to a food.

What is a food intolerance?

A food intolerance is a symptomatic reaction to a food or food component that is generally less severe than a food allergy. A food intolerance occurs when:

- the body lacks a particular enzyme to digest nutrients (such as lactase, the enzyme required to digest lactose, the sugar in milk)
- nutrients are too abundant to be properly digested
- a particular nutrient cannot be digested sufficiently.[1]

Symptoms of food intolerance are mostly related to the digestive system and tend to occur after gut bacteria ferment a food, leading to the production of gas, which can trigger abdominal pain, bloating and irregular bowel movements. Often, this happens because of an enzyme deficiency. In other cases, the gut may simply have a hard time breaking nutrients down, particularly if you've consumed a large portion of food in one sitting!

The symptoms of food intolerance usually take longer to emerge compared with food allergies – several hours and even up to three days after eating the trigger food.

Unlike food allergies, food intolerances are often dose-related, which means that symptoms may only be experienced when eating a large portion of the offending food or if it is eaten very frequently. For example, a person with lactose intolerance might get away with drinking a splash of milk in their morning coffee but become unwell when they drink a pint of milk.

In some cases, a whole food group can cause trouble, but it is also possible to be intolerant to just one or two foods within a group. For example, someone might be able to tolerate cheese but not milk or yoghurt.

Common examples of food intolerances include lactose or fructose intolerance, as well as intolerance to other FODMAPs (see p. 126).

Other intolerances and CFS

Histamine is a substance produced in the body and released in response to an injury or allergic reaction. It is also found in many foods, such as avocados, tomatoes, dried fruits and fermented foods (for example sauerkraut and some alcoholic beverages). While not strictly speaking a food intolerance, this intolerance occurs when histamine builds up in the body faster than it can be broken down, often due to a deficiency of an enzyme called diamine oxidase (DAO). Histamine intolerance can be common in CFS patients who have problems with the functioning of their mast cells, resulting in symptoms that mirror CFS.

Then there is sulphur intolerance. Sulphur is an essential

mineral in the diet, involved in, among other functions, methylation processes and detoxification. Sulphur is found in protein-rich foods such as meat, cheese and fish, as well as plant-based sources, such as cruciferous vegetables, garlic, onions and beans. Despite the importance of sulphur's role in the body, problems can often stem from an inability to keep it in balance, and, when it starts to build up in the body, it can lead to symptoms that align with CFS. This can be driven by a high intake of sulphur-rich foods (although it would be impossible to avoid it in the diet completely), as well as by issues breaking down and metabolising sulphur in the body (these can be related to genetic SNPs, dysbiosis or SIBO in the gut).

Note: sulphur intolerance is not the same as sulphite reactions, which can result from the additives commonly used in food preservation (as in winemaking, for example).

What is a food sensitivity?

Often, the terms food intolerance and food sensitivity are used interchangeably; however, there is a difference between the two. A food sensitivity is an immune-mediated reaction to a food that, just like intolerances, can give rise to digestive symptoms; but they can also cause widespread symptoms (known as extra-intestinal symptoms), such as fatigue, brain fog, headaches, sinus problems, fluid retention, joint pain and skin rashes. Like intolerances, food sensitivities can also have a delayed onset.

In food sensitivity, the immune system has lost its ability to tolerate food proteins via the gut, driving inflammation within the body (this is known as a loss of oral tolerance). Silent inflammation can occur through an autoimmune process called molecular mimicry, which is when an invader (in this case, a food protein) enters the bloodstream (often through a leaky gut) and the immune system starts to attack the body's own tissues in a case of mistaken identity. It can make this error when bodily tissues hold a similar molecular structure to what is considered to be an invader (in this case a food protein) and, if there is a propensity towards autoimmunity, it erroneously starts to mount an inflammatory response. It might be brain tissue, the small intestine (as in coeliac disease, when gluten is consumed) or the thyroid that gets caught up in the crossfire, and this process can go undetected for years and years, until symptoms start to present themselves. Eventually, this could lead to the development of autoimmune disease.

Scientists have recently identified a phenomenon called non-coeliac gluten sensitivity (NCGS), which is thought to sit under this umbrella of food sensitivity (see p. 139 for more on this).

Was it just a food reaction all along?

It seems more plausible to accept that a peanut can cause swelling of the lips and throat than that the milk or bread you consume is triggering your CFS symptoms. However, it is important not to disregard the possibility of food intolerance or sensitivity, and the idea that eliminating a food from your diet may result in an improvement in your symptoms.

It may have been the case that you were suffering with food reactions *before* you became unwell with CFS and that these have worsened with the illness. However, the most likely scenario is that food intolerances and sensitivities may be a *symptom* of CFS and a part of your overall clinical picture – the rationale being that if the digestive, nervous and immune systems are all dysregulated, you are highly likely to see food reactions arise as a result. That's why removing any potential problem foods from your diet can grant the body some much needed relief, allowing time to repair and restore.

Note: symptoms of food sensitivity and intolerance may be caused by other conditions, so make sure that you communicate all your symptoms to your GP, so that alternative explanations are ruled out before proceeding with any dietary protocols.

Identifying a food intolerance or sensitivity

It can be hard to spot intolerances or sensitivities to certain foods, especially if symptoms have a delayed onset.

Also, food intolerances and sensitivities can be hidden, as well as fixed or variable. If they are fixed, you will have a reaction every single time you come into contact with the food in question; if they are variable, other factors need to be present alongside the food – such as stress, menstruation (women), hormonal fluctuations, portion size, how the food is eaten – to elicit a response in the body. In other scenarios, it may be food combining that causes problems – for instance, you may do just fine with strawberries, and do well with yoghurt, but not with strawberries and yoghurt together in the same meal.

What's more, symptoms of food reactivity can go completely unnoticed, as you start to adapt to the reactions. This is because you may have forgotten what it feels like to feel fully well and therefore symptoms go undetected. Or, as we have established with food sensitivity, there may not be any noticeable symptoms initially, but silent inflammation is occurring (which could lead to symptoms appearing over time).

There are multiple tests on the market that claim to 'diagnose' your food reactions via a simple blood or skin-prick test. However, the efficacy of some of these tests is sometimes disputed, with false positive and negative results often reported.

Therefore, food-reactivity testing can be an added expense to your recovery budget, which can backfire if you do not select an appropriate test. Therefore, the method I most commonly turn to when assessing whether someone has a food intolerance or sensitivity is a slightly more laborious process involving an elimination diet, followed by a structured reintroduction of the food(s) in question.

The elimination diet
In my clinical practice, I use elimination diets to identify food reactions using a three-stage approach:

- The food-monitoring phase
- The elimination phase
- The reintroduction-challenge (provocation) phase

1. **Food-monitoring phase** Complete a three-week food and symptom diary, which will help you to identify any trigger foods or food

components that may be related to your symptoms. (You must note down every single thing you consume, no matter how small.) Score each of your daily symptoms out of 6 (0 being the best and 6 being the worst), while taking into consideration portion size, as well as lifestyle factors, such as stress, hormonal shifts (such as menstruation), eating on the go, etc. Once you have isolated any potential problem foods, move on to the next stage. See my example of a food-and-symptom diary on the next page.

2. **Elimination phase** Once you have identified any suspected trigger food(s) or food components, the next phase involves eliminating them from your diet for a minimum of six weeks. At the end of the allotted time, assess whether you have observed a clear improvement in your symptoms. If you have noticed an improvement, you can progress to stage 3, the reintroduction-challenge phase. If you have not seen any change, it may be worth checking whether you have succeeded in fully removing the suspected food(s) or food components from your diet. Remember that ingredients can be hidden in packaged foods such as sauces and dressings, and may have initially gone unnoticed, so read nutrition labels very carefully. Aim to consume foods in their natural state, rather than raiding the 'free from' aisle. In some cases, you may need to continue with the elimination phase for a little longer to see if symptoms start to lessen over time.

Do also be aware of cross-contamination, which is where food proteins that you are trying to avoid accidentally end up in your meal due to food preparation (via shared utensils or food surfaces) or manufacturing processes.

If you have succeeded in being stringent and have removed the suspected problem foods for the six-week period (or longer) but are still experiencing symptoms, you may not be intolerant or sensitive to those foods or food components after all. Progress on to the reintroduction-challenge phase to test how the foods impact your body when reintroduced. You can always return to the food-monitoring phase and follow the process again by isolating any other suspected trigger foods, in the hope of identifying another possible offender.

	Monday	Tuesday	Wednesday
Breakfast	Bowl of low-sugar cereal with oat milk and sliced pear	Porridge with sliced banana and pumpkin seeds	Homemade granola with oat milk and cherries
Snack			Half an orange
Lunch	Two vegetarian sausages, rocket and tomatoes in pita bread	Poké bowl with smoked salmon and edamame	Carrot and coriander soup with oat biscuits
Snack	Pack of salt and vinegar crisps		
Dinner	Whole wheat pasta with tomato and mascarpone sauce with grated Cheddar cheese	Tofu and rice vermicelli noodle stir fry with sweetcorn, edamame, onions, pak choi, red pepper, and tamari sauce	Cheese and tomato pizza with rocket and sliced olives
Snack		Apple	
Drinks	2–3l water with lime cordial throughout the day	2–3l water Glass of orange juice Green tea	2l water with cucumber infusion Green tea
Symptoms score (/6)	Didn't notice a change in my symptoms, felt quite good (fatigue, brain fog and gut symptoms are all 0/6). Stress levels relatively normal. Larger portion sizes than usual (second helpings at dinner).	Woke up this morning and the bloating was back (5/6). I think this was the cheese and pasta I had last night because it didn't sit right in my gut all evening (I did eat a large portion of it, too). Brain fog symptoms are 3/6 and fatigue symptoms are 2/6.	Gut symptoms improved today (2/6), brain fog still at 3/6 and fatigue is still 2/6. Argument with partner this evening. Overly anxious and worried about health.

Thursday	Friday	Saturday	Sunday
No breakfast		Two poached eggs, one sausage, steamed spinach and baked beans	Ham, mushroom and tomato omelette
Two fried eggs on two slices of buttered wholegrain toast	Carrot and coriander soup with oat crackers	Leftover prawn and rocket salad	Chicken and roasted pepper stew with celery and onion
Raspberries and strawberries			
Two vegetarian burgers with mixed vegetables and oven chips	Prawn and rocket salad with sliced mango, bell pepper, spring onion and lime juice	Lamb kebabs served with houmous, tzakiki and baba ganoush	Roast beef with horseradish, carrot, roast potatoes and broccoli with gravy
Three chocolate digestive biscuits		One bowl of popcorn	Small bowl of grapes
2l water 2 glasses of wine	1.5l water	2l water	5 glasses of water
Gut symptoms are worse today. I can notice an association between how I feel and the pizza I ate last night. I also realised I had a stressful day yesterday and ate on the go, which I think has worsened the abdominal discomfort and bloating (5/6). Brain fog symptoms 4/6 and fatigue 5/6.	Still feeling slightly off this morning (fatigue 4/6, brain fog 4/6, bloating 5/6). Symptoms starting to settle down this afternoon. More of a relaxed day today and the onset of the weekend providing me with time to rest is brightening my mood.	Woke up feeling a little more refreshed after more sleep and a lie-in. Brain fog has improved to 2/6, Bloating has reduced to 2/6 and fatigue is 2/6.	Feeling similar to yesterday but appreciative that symptoms have not worsened. Brain fog 2/6, bloating 2/6 and fatigue 2/6.

Give it a go at home using the template below:

	Monday	Tuesday	Wednesday
Breakfast			
Snack			
Lunch			
Snack			
Dinner			
Snack			
Drinks			
Symptoms score (/6)			

Thursday	Friday	Saturday	Sunday

3. **Reintroduction-challenge (provocation) phase** This is about reintroducing the foods or food components that were eliminated, with the goal of assessing whether eating them again causes symptoms to reappear. Start by reintroducing the foods (one at a time, if multiple foods were eliminated) to observe any reactions. For each food that you reintroduce, wait a period of three days before bringing back any others, so that any delayed reaction is not open to misinterpretation.

    Reintroduce foods gradually, starting with one or two average-sized portions (say, a cup of yoghurt or two eggs), while continuing to eat the foods you are permitted. Continue completing your food and symptom diary to establish whether the reintroduced food is tolerated or not. If a food causes a reaction, you should eliminate it again and wait until symptoms subside before reintroducing any other foods. You can retest the foods that give you symptoms after you have tested all your other challenge foods, using the same process of waiting three days for a response and using your food and symptom diary for tracking. If a reintroduced food *still* gives you symptoms, eliminate it for three to six months and then reassess with a healthcare practitioner.

    If a food that is reintroduced produces no reaction, then try out a new one after three days (this might be a food from the same family as the one you reintroduced previously – for example Manchego cheese after the introduction of yoghurt). If there is no reaction, keep that food in your diet, introduce the next challenge food and so on.

This process certainly requires patience, but it is the best way of observing how well your body responds to particular foods, helping you to gather feedback and get to know your body and its symptoms. Further support can be gained by working closely with a practitioner if you are struggling to do this alone.

Top tip: a bowl of pasta on its own is a lot easier to track symptoms against than a lasagne containing both dairy and gluten, for example. It's also best to avoid reintroducing foods in situations that make it difficult to interpret results, such as when you are feeling unwell due to stress, a poor night's sleep or an infection. Reintroduce foods at a time where you feel relatively stable, and when your symptoms are not rapidly fluctuating for other non-food-related reasons.

The AIP diet

If you don't have time to follow the food-monitoring phase and would prefer to jump in feet first, another option is to try something called the autoimmune protocol diet (AIP) for a minimum of six weeks. This is essentially a paleo diet with a few additional restrictions on foods that may trigger symptoms. It means no grains (including pseudograins – buckwheat, quinoa and amaranth, for example), no legumes (beans, lentils, peas, peanuts), no dairy and nothing refined or ultra-processed, as well as no eggs, nuts, seeds and vegetables from the nightshade family (potatoes, tomatoes, aubergines, peppers), nor alcohol and coffee. The focus is on a diet of organ and grass-fed meats (organically sourced, where possible), seafood (wild-caught) and as many vegetables as possible (besides nightshades), along with fermented foods and bone broth. Fruit is permitted in moderation.

This diet allows time for the gut to repair and calm down any inflammation. However, the drawback is that it can be very difficult to stick to and is heavily restrictive, so it is not for everyone (especially not vegans or vegetarians). Also, if followed for too long, the AIP diet can lead to nutrient deficiencies, so always seek the support of a qualified nutritional practitioner if you are looking to explore this route.

After six weeks on the AIP diet (and depending on how well you feel), you can gradually begin to reintroduce foods, following the same steps as in the reintroduction-challenge phase of the elimination diet (see above) to see whether symptoms are triggered and if there are any food reactions.

Note: if you have an eating disorder (or a history of one), do not attempt to remove foods from your diet and please seek professional one-to-one support regarding your nutrition.

If I'm intolerant or sensitive to a food, do I need to avoid it for life?

Our ability to tolerate certain foods can alter over time (particularly as our microbiome, immune and hormonal profiles change).

By taking problem foods out of the diet for long enough, your body (namely the gut and immune system) gain a breather and a chance to repair and rebalance. There may then come a time when you can go back to eating those foods again in normal, but perhaps not excessive quantities.

With intolerance and sensitivity, there is more scope to experiment with problem foods and see whether other factors are at play, as opposed to food allergy, where you may need to avoid the problem food for life to remain symptom-free.

In the majority of cases, food intolerances and sensitivities should not mean having to exclude things for ever, unless they still cause you trouble when you reintroduce them. The idea is to experiment and, ultimately, to find a tailormade diet that suits you and your physiology in the long run.

For my clients with histamine, sulphur or FODMAP intolerance, I ask them to minimise high-histamine, high-sulphur or high-FODMAP foods if they are becoming an issue. I find that people tend not to take issue with the word 'minimise', as opposed to a blanket restriction, which many find more difficult.

The gluten conundrum

Gluten-free or not gluten-free? That is the question . . .

Gluten-containing foods are heavily woven into the fabric of the Western diet in breads, pasta, pizza, biscuits, pastry and cakes, to name a few. There is considerable anecdotal evidence in support of going gluten-free for CFS recovery. Certainly, this was part of my own journey. However, is this simply a trend, since gluten-free diets are all the rage right now, or does it have any scientific validity when it comes to improvement in CFS symptoms?

Before we go any further, what exactly is gluten?

Gluten is a family of proteins found in grains such as wheat, barley and rye. Oats do not naturally contain gluten; however, in some manufacturing processes, they can be cross-contaminated.

The wheat we eat today is not the same as it was thousands of years ago, as modern farming practices have produced a version with a much higher gluten content.

What's more, glyphosate (a weedkiller, also known as RoundUp) is a common pesticide used to treat land that grows wheat and barley, which we know is detrimental to the gut microbiome. So it's fair to say that as a population we are consuming a lot more gluten today than ever before, along with a significant proportion of harmful pesticides, too.

Individual gluten tolerance may be a question of how the grains are prepared, so considerations regarding the overall quality of wheat and gluten should come into question. Sourdough is an example of a fermented source, where some of the gluten content is broken down, making it more tolerable for some. If you do not have gluten sensitivity, and your body can handle it, it's preferable to opt for organic and ancient grains such as einkorn, emmer and spelt. When it comes to bread, the longer the panification (bread-making) process, the better it is at reducing gluten content, so do ask questions when purchasing your bread.

You may have heard of coeliac disease (CD), an autoimmune condition that causes damage to the lining of the small intestine when gluten is eaten. It affects 1 in 100 people in the UK and is on the rise, with an estimated half a million people going undiagnosed. Then there is wheat allergy (WA), a traditional food allergy that causes a severe immune response whenever wheat is consumed.

Scientists are also on the cusp of understanding what they have termed gluten-related disorders. One example is non-coeliac gluten sensitivity (NCGS), which is defined as a sensitivity to gluten in the absence of a CD or WA diagnosis. Studies have linked NCGS with digestive symptoms, as well as widespread symptoms that are hallmarks of CFS, including fatigue, brain fog, vertigo and dizziness. There are currently no tests to diagnose NCGS, so the condition is currently confirmed by the onset of symptoms following gluten consumption and symptom improvement following a gluten-free diet, after ruling out WA and CD.

There is also evidence that demonstrates the benefits of following a gluten-free diet on reducing thyroid antibodies in Hashimoto's disease[2], as well as supporting other non-coeliac autoimmune conditions.[3]

Note: if you suspect that you have a problem with gluten, the first thing to do before removing it from your diet is to get tested for coeliac disease. This is very important because gluten must have been consumed for a period of six weeks before testing to obtain a positive coeliac-disease test result.

Gluten and leaky gut

While understanding of intestinal permeability and its associations with chronic disease (including CFS) is still in its infancy, there is evidence linking gluten consumption with a leaky gut.[4] (It might interest you to know that this is applicable to *everybody* who consumes gluten, and not just exclusively those with CD or NCGS.)

In those with autoimmune conditions and gluten-related disorders such as NCGS (which may overlap with CFS), the inflammatory load of eating gluten can start to become a real health burden. I have had CFS clients who have been able to eradicate symptoms (and some have even lowered their levels of autoimmune antibodies) by adopting a gluten-free diet, so it is certainly worth consideration if you are at a fork in the road when it comes to recovery and reducing inflammation. Plus, it can be used as a preventative tool to help ward off future autoimmune diseases (which can be helpful if your CFS has some autoimmune origin).

A two-way street

Food sensitivities (to gluten, for example) can cause a leaky gut, while having a leaky gut can also make us more susceptible to developing food sensitivities (see also p. 76).

Eliminating gluten: pros and cons

Life isn't black or white; it's all sorts of shades of grey and everything else in between. When it comes to gluten, how much you need to avoid it and for how long will depend entirely on you, and how you respond to the elimination diet on pp. 130–136, as well as how well you can support the integrity of your gut lining through the 5R approach (more of which on p. 144). This is where the concept of bio-individuality comes into play.

Naturally, there are those who believe that going gluten-free is not such a healthy choice. This is because many people who follow gluten-free diets tend to avoid most grains, which provide a wealth of nutrients, including B vitamins (vital for energy production) and, most importantly, fibre. However, a variety of gluten-free grains, such as teff, millet and sorghum, are among the many other B-vitamin and fibre-rich alternatives available to those on gluten-free diets.

It's also argued that gluten-free diets are high in 'free-from' junk foods that are nutritionally depleted and high in sugars and unhealthy fats. However, it is certainly possible to avoid these processed alternatives by opting for gluten-free whole foods instead.

There is also some evidence that removing gluten from the diet can diminish the diversity of friendly bacteria in the microbiome (again, due to the lack-of-fibre argument), which is why I advise feeding your microbiome with a diverse array of plant fibres to get around this if you do opt to go gluten-free.

Overall, going gluten-free is unlikely to do you any harm in terms of nutritional deficiencies, providing you get sufficient fibre from other foods and nurture your microbiome through dietary diversity.

Long term, depending on how your body handles gluten when it is reintroduced, I believe that in most cases it is ultimately a question of quality and quantity. Many of us consume gluten in every meal, so lowering your gluten consumption certainly wouldn't hurt and you can also be doing yourself some favours in fighting the inflammation battle.

Ultimately, quantifying the need to adopt a gluten-free diet for CFS in the absence of CD is a personal cost–benefit exercise. Moreover, your relationship with food can certainly come into consideration here, too (more on this on p. 176). Therefore, while we certainly need more studies to understand the clinical application of gluten-free diets in CFS to support dietary speculations, it's a question of:

- what the gut can deal with
- what the immune system can deal with
- how tolerance can be restored to achieve an inclusive, diverse diet overall.

Restrictive diets are always meant to be short term, the overarching goal being to expand the variety of foods that you eat. It is also important to understand that food isn't the entire problem; food reactions are often symptoms of a greater dysregulation and, once addressed, tolerance (and symptoms) can start to improve.

I have had clients who have received diagnoses of CFS and fibromyalgia, and who, having undertaken food-and-symptom diaries, were able to isolate gluten and dairy as trigger foods. My recommendation was that they first rule out coeliac disease with a test from the GP, and then, in the event that it was negative, follow an elimination diet. The goal then was to rebuild their diets to allow for inclusivity and diversity, based on their improved health and gut tolerance over time.

The jury is still out and there are some competing theories surrounding where the problem lies besides solely blaming gluten when it comes to those with medically unexplained syndromes, including CFS and IBS. There are other compounds in gluten and wheat-containing foods that are also up for debate; some fingers point towards FODMAPs, amylase trypsin inhibitors (ATIs) or wheat germ agglutinin. Therefore, more research is needed to widen our knowledge further.

Ditch the dairy?

Dairy products are foods or beverages produced from the milk of mammals, such as cow's milk, cheese, butter, yoghurt and cream. (**Note:** this does not include eggs.)

Along with gluten, dairy is another common offender when it comes to food intolerance and sensitivity. It appears that while lactose intolerance is a problem for approximately 65 per cent of the world's population, many people can also have a sensitivity to the proteins found in dairy products, namely casein and whey.

On the surface, dairy is a nourishing food group. It contains a good dose of protein, calcium and fat-soluble nutrients, such as vitamins A, D, E and K. Additionally, full-fat dairy contains compounds that have protective effects on the gut lining, such as butyrate. However, most of our milk today is pasteurised (a process of heating milk to very high temperatures to kill off any harmful bacteria and increase shelf life), which is great if you're pregnant, but pasteurisation doesn't discriminate, which means that any beneficial bacteria, vitamins and enzymes are also wiped out in the process.

It's also common practice for milk to be homogenised – a process that aims to break down the fat globules into smaller components, helping it to disperse evenly – but again, this can also destroy vital vitamins and minerals, while reducing the size and composition of the fat molecules in a way that makes it easier for them to enter the bloodstream, potentially carrying unwanted health risks.

For those who do choose to consume dairy, organic is always best, since dairy foods repeatedly top the list of foods containing harmful pesticides, antibiotics and synthetic hormones. Of all the dairy products, yoghurt, kefir and quark are some of the better options for gut health (in particular, for those with lactose intolerance), since they are fermented, which breaks down the lactose content, while packing in some probiotics in the process.

For some, it may be worth eliminating dairy in the initial stages of CFS to see how your symptoms respond. This may also offer some benefit for those CFS patients who are gluten sensitive (NCGS) and not experiencing symptom relief on a gluten-free diet alone. It's always worth a try to see how you feel.

A client of mine who was suffering with CFS also received a diagnosis of Hashimoto's thyroiditis. I recommended removing gluten from her diet and reducing her consumption of conventional dairy products, while supporting her thyroid and gut through nutritional measures in the process. The elimination approach helped to lower inflammation in her body, and we were able to reduce her thyroid antibody levels as a result.

In the long run, you decide. Dairy doesn't necessarily have to be off limits for ever if you have CFS – just don't make it a mainstay of your diet. And if you do happen to tolerate a bit of dairy, go for full-fat, or otherwise avoid the highly processed low-fat dairy with added sugars and thickening agents. Sheep's and goat's milk might also be better options for those who are dairy sensitive, since they contain the protein beta-casein a2 (most cow's milk contains beta-casein a1, which more people are prone to reacting to).

Now that we have established a case for exploring an elimination diet for CFS, let's look at this within the framework of my 5R plan, which aims to bolster the health of the gut and work towards physiological balance.

The 5R Plan

As we saw in Part 2, the gut is the intersection of the various body systems that play a role in energy production, as well as being a likely driver of many CFS symptoms. It is, therefore, one of the key routes to resolving CFS.

The aim of the game is to create a flourishing microbiome and deal with any imbalances identified within the digestive tract (such as infections, dysbiosis and inflammation), that, in turn, can feed into the various other chronic stressors that may form part of your CFS picture.

My 5R plan – Remove, Replace, Reinoculate, Repair, Rebalance – will start you on the road to restoring your health:

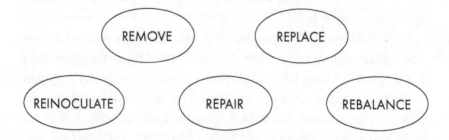

1. Remove

This stage is all about removing any unruly foods and pathogens that may be fanning the flames of dysbiosis and chronic inflammation within your gut and compounding fatigue symptoms. To support your recovery from CFS, look to avoid (or limit) the following (and non-CFS sufferers could benefit from doing this, too!):

- Free sugars and refined carbohydrates
- Ultra-processed foods
- Artificial sweeteners and sugar alcohols
- Caffeine
- Alcohol
- Trans fats
- Soya

Let's look at each of these in a little more detail.

Free sugars and refined carbohydrates
The Western diet is renowned for foods that are high in sugar (think biscuits, cakes, croissants, cereals, white bread, pastries, chocolate, sweetened fizzy beverages). These make for a highly inflammatory and weight-gaining diet that wreaks havoc on our energy, hormones, gut bacteria and immune system.

But when we talk about sugar, what do we mean?

Before we go any further, let's explore carbohydrates, aka 'carbs'. It is worth knowing that not all carbs are created equally. The three main types are sugars, starches and fibre. They are called 'simple' or 'complex', based on their chemical make-up and what your body does with them.

Simple carbs are composed of one or two easy-to-digest sugar molecules (known as monosaccharides and disaccharides). Some of these are naturally occurring, such as those found in fruits (fructose) or milk (lactose). They are also found in refined sugars, such as 'table sugar', which contains sucrose. (**Note:** sucrose can also be found naturally in maple syrup and coconut sugar.) Simple carbs are also found in grains that have been refined to remove their fibrous bran (for example, white bread or flour or white pasta and rice).

Starch is a complex carbohydrate found naturally in many grains, pulses and vegetables – think corn, peas, potatoes, kidney beans, parsnips and sweet potatoes. They consist of longer chains of sugar molecules (polysaccharides), which the body slowly breaks down into glucose – the body's preferred source of energy.

Fibre is another type of complex carbohydrate, but it passes through the digestive system unchanged, and our gut bugs love the stuff – it is a food source for our friendly gut bacteria, and it also slows the rate of digestion of other carbohydrates (including starches and simple sugars), making it excellent for blood-sugar control.

Refined-sugar foods tend to be lacking in fibre, which means that they spike our blood-sugar levels at a much quicker rate than usual, taxing the health of our adrenal glands. They have also been associated with creating an environment for disruptive microbes in the gut to thrive.

What's more, whenever we eat refined-sugar foods, our blood-sugar levels start to rise, triggering the pancreas to release a hormone called insulin that helps the body's cells utilise this sugar for energy. Raised blood-sugar levels can lead to something called glycation, where proteins and fats bind together with sugar in the bloodstream to form advanced glycation end products (AGEs) – powerful pro-oxidants that can cause an internal rusting that damages cells and body tissues. AGEs are thought to be involved in chronic diseases such as CFS, contributing to inflammation and even the ageing process.

When blood-sugar levels get too high, we tend to experience a rapid surge of energy, which is soon followed by a crash in energy. This 'blood-sugar rollercoaster' is all too familiar to many people with CFS – those dreaded feelings of fatigue throughout the day, compounded by the highs and lows of sugar consumption and dependency.

When blood-sugar levels drop, it also causes physical stress on the body. Cortisol levels go up when blood sugar goes down, helping to raise your blood sugar to a normal level again. If you have blood-sugar imbalances, you could be compounding adrenal issues in order to regulate blood sugar.

The word 'sugar' broadly refers to the following:

- Sugars that are naturally occurring and bound within the cellular structure of many foods, such as fructose in fruit or lactose in milk.

- Sugars that are added to food or drink by manufacturers or during the cooking process. These are the types that we can most easily spot and reduce in our diet and are known as 'free sugars'. Our daily consumption of free sugars should be less than 5 per cent of our total energy intake (which is no more than seven teaspoons of sugar daily). And remember, this is a limit and not necessarily a target! Examples of free sugars include:
  - refined sugar, often referred to as 'table sugar' and added to various foods and desserts, or cups of tea or coffee
  - honey, coconut sugar, maple syrup, and high-fructose corn syrup (**note:** these also come under the sweetener category)
  - pure fruit juice – because the fructose has been separated from the fibre within the fruit.

- Natural or artificial sweeteners. Natural sweeteners include sugar alcohols such as sorbitol, xylitol and mannitol; honey, maple syrup and coconut sugar (**note:** while these are classed as natural sweeteners, they can still be somewhat processed). Artificial sweeteners include aspartame, saccharin, sucralose, high-fructose corn syrup.

To balance your blood sugar, try to make wise choices, avoiding free sugars and refined carbohydrates and instead opting for slower-releasing ('complex') carbohydrates, which are digested much more slowly. Complex-carb foods include wholegrains, legumes and starchy vegetables, such as sweet potato or squash. Try to pair your sources of carbs with protein- and fibre-rich foods.

Be ingredients savvy

Start looking more carefully at the labels on your food packaging. As a rule of thumb, if the first ingredient is sugar (or any derivative that can typically end with the suffix 'ose' – 'glucose', 'maltose', 'dextrose') or syrup (including 'cane sugar syrup', for instance), that food is likely to be high in sugar. This is because ingredients are listed in descending order based on their quantities – so the higher up on the list, the more of it there is. Also, look for the carbohydrate content. A low-sugar food would typically have less than 5g total sugars per 100g, versus a high-sugar food that contains more than 22.5g of total sugars per 100g.

Ultra-processed foods

The term 'processed food' gets a bad rap, but all the food we eat is processed to some degree – grains are milled into flour, fish is tinned and vegetables can be frozen. Food processing can help to preserve and transform food, making it last for much longer.

In the last fifty years, however, we have seen a rise in novel food-processing techniques that can negatively influence our health. Foods that have undergone such processes are termed 'ultra-processed foods' and have been associated with lowered immunity, reduced microbiome diversity, gut inflammation and chronic disease.

Minimally processed and natural foods	Cooking ingredients	Processed foods	Ultra-processed foods
Corn	Butter	Tinned mackerel	Carrot cake
Apple	Honey	Salted peanuts	Corn chips
Salmon	Salt	Tinned chickpeas	Fizzy lemonade
Eggs	Sugar	Bacon	Margarine
Broccoli	Maple syrup	Freshly made feta	Cereal bar
Potato	Olive oil	Wine	Microwavable pizza

Try to focus on positive nutrition, buying foods in their natural state that are not boxed, bagged, heavily manipulated or masquerading as something that they are not.

Artificial sweeteners and sugar alcohols

It's easy to believe that artificial sweeteners are a perfect replacement for our societal sugar addiction, especially when they are low- or zero-calorie and many aren't counted as part of our 'free-sugar' intake, but one of the problems with many of these is that they can wreak havoc on the gut microbiome, depleting beneficial communities of bugs. They can also spell trouble for the metabolism and nervous system, which isn't the best combination if you have CFS.

In comparison, many natural sweeteners are high in sugar alcohols (polyols), which are a type of FODMAP (see p. 126), so they are not properly absorbed in the small intestine. As a result, they travel to the large intestine where they are fermented by gut bacteria, causing gas, bloating and many other digestive symptoms. And if the digestive system is in distress, feelings of fatigue will worsen as a result.

My advice is to avoid artificial sweeteners and sugar alcohols altogether.

Caffeine

Caffeine is one of the world's most used drugs. It increases activity in certain parts of the brain and central nervous system. And it stimulates the adrenal glands to trigger adrenaline and cortisol, causing the physical effects involved in the 'fight-or-flight' response (i.e. an initial surge of energy).

Chronic caffeine consumption can wreak havoc on energy levels, due to its effect on one of our brain chemicals (adenosine), and people can become caffeine dependent, needing more and more of it just to function 'normally'.

Just like sugar, caffeine feeds the blood-sugar rollercoaster, compounding feelings of fatigue and HPA-axis dysfunction. It can also interfere with vitamin and mineral absorption, including water-soluble B vitamins, which we so heavily rely on for energy. This means that caffeine can make fatigue much worse, particularly if you are sensitive to its effects.

If you don't feel the adverse effects of coffee, stick to no more than two cups a day and no later than 2pm (caffeine has a six-hour half-life, which means it takes approximately that long for half of it to be metabolised and leave the body – so if you are drinking coffee past 2pm, you could be in for a restless night's sleep). I'm not suggesting everyone with CFS should quit caffeine completely (although some people may feel that's the best option for them), but do be mindful of your consumption. Oh, and if you do have the odd cup of Joe, make sure you go for organic, as coffee beans tend to rank high among the crops most sprayed with pesticides.

Decaffeinated coffees are also an option, although a lot of these use chemicals to remove the caffeine, so try to choose clean decaf brands or try alternatives, such as chicory 'coffee' or herbal/fruit teas.

Remember: caffeine is also in chocolate, energy drinks, cola and some herbal teas (green tea, for example). Always check the labels.

Alcohol

The health hazards of alcohol are numerous and, since many CFS patients struggle with alcohol intolerance, it is an obvious one to rule out to support long-term health and recovery.

Alcohol is known to deplete gut bacteria and incite a leaky gut. It leads to blood-sugar issues, lowers immunity, taxes the liver and adrenals and encourages oxidative stress. Drinking alcohol can also reduce absorption of B vitamins, which are critical in the production of energy. So a teetotal period, particularly if you are in the most difficult stage of your illness, is certainly a sensible move. Saying goodbye to booze and hello to H_2O can support detoxification processes, helping to catapult the body into a recovery state.

Also, contrary to popular belief, those little nightcaps that people think will help them to relax and sleep more soundly actually interfere with sleep quality by suppressing production of melatonin (a hormone that plays a key role in regulating circadian rhythm – aka your 'biological clock'), causing next-day tiredness and fatigue.

Trans fats

Trans fats are fats that have been hydrogenated, a process designed to prolong shelf life.

These types of fats have been linked with heart disease and diabetes, as well as chronic inflammation. Since we don't want to be adding fuel to the fire when it comes to inflammation in CFS, trans fats should be avoided at all costs for the benefit of your long-term health and wellbeing.

Importantly, unlike the artificial trans fats you see in margarines, baked goods and ultra-processed foods, natural forms occurring in animal products (such as red meat and dairy) are not considered harmful if consumed in moderate amounts.

Soya

Soya is a controversial food, due to its high isoflavone content. It is a plant compound that can mimic the effects of oestrogen in the body (it is known as a phytoestrogen). The isoflavones in soya can also be classified as goitrogens, which are compounds that interfere with thyroid function.

None the less, the soya bean is a fantastic source of plant-based protein, offering all the essential amino acids required for vegetarians and vegans. To find some middle ground, I always recommend that those with CFS who have thyroid dysfunction (or iodine deficiency) limit their soya intake to no more than twice a week, avoiding processed soya and opting instead for quality sources that are organic and fermented, like miso and tempeh, so that the body assimilates its components much better (although do watch out for soya if you are histamine intolerant). If you are on thyroid medication, always ensure that any soya is consumed either four hours before or after you take it (because it can interfere with your medication's absorption).

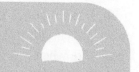

Dealing with dysbiosis: 'weed out' the bad bugs

The removal stage also involves dealing with any pathogens detected in functional tests (such as pathogenic bacteria, yeasts, parasites or viruses), which may be fuelling CFS symptoms. This may warrant the use of anti-microbial supplements such as:

Oil of oregano	Extracted from the leaves of the oregano herb, oil of oregano contains two powerful compounds called carvacrol and thymol, which have been shown to exhibit natural antibacterial, antifungal, antiviral and antiparasitic properties. I often find oil of oregano useful in the case of dysbiosis, wherever there is an overgrowth of bacteria in the small or large intestine.
Grapefruit seed extract	Sometimes referred to as 'citricidal', grapefruit seed extract is great for fighting bacterial and fungal dysbiosis. Plus, it contains naringenin, an antioxidant to protect the body against free radicals.
Caprylic acid	A medium chain fatty acid (MCT) found in coconuts, caprylic acid is a go-to natural supplement when there is a yeast infection (i.e. overgrowth of Candida albicans); it has been shown to fight against these microorganisms. It also has antibacterial properties.
Wormwood	Prized for its compound thujone, wormwood is a herb that is often combined with black walnut and clove to help in breaking the life cycle of parasites.
Elderberry extract	Also known as Sambucus nigra, elderberry is an antioxidant-rich fruit with various benefits for health. The extract has been used medicinally for centuries to help fight viruses, with some studies showing its promise in fighting influenza viruses.[5] Many of these benefits are attributed to compounds called anthocyanins – phytochemicals in the elderberry that provide its vivid purple colour.

Japanese knotweed	Japanese knotweed is a plant containing a polyphenol called resveratrol. Its constituents have been shown to cross the blood–brain barrier and act as an anti-inflammatory agent in the brain and central nervous system. Studies have also shown some promise in working well against the bacteria that causes Lyme disease (Borrelia burgdorferi).[6]
Black walnut	Black walnut comes from a tree of the same name. The tannins in black walnuts harness antibacterial properties. Black walnut can also be used for parasitic infections, and there is also some evidence that it can help to fight Borrelia burgdorferi (the bacteria that causes Lyme disease).[7]

The weeding process may take some time and will depend on what each individual has going on within their unique ecosystem. Of course, not everybody with CFS will require this approach, but anti-microbial agents can certainly be a useful tool if infections and/or dysbiosis have been identified as a prominent concern.

Note: please do not supplement without consulting a healthcare professional, and always disclose all medications that you are currently taking, due to the potential risk of drug/nutrient interactions.

EMILY, AGED TWENTY-SEVEN

At the age of twenty-five, I was diagnosed with CFS. My main symptom was severe fatigue, but I also experienced a variety of debilitating digestive issues, particularly bloating.

I went to see Lauren and she ran a stool test with me, which uncovered the presence of a parasite in my digestive system, as well as dysbiosis (an overgrowth of pathogenic bacteria and yeast), which meant that my gut was inflamed and under a considerable amount of stress.

I followed a 5R protocol as part of Lauren's recommendations, removing high-sugar and ultra-processed foods from my diet, while 'weeding' to balance the ecology of my gut, using some natural anti-microbial agents (including wormwood, black walnut and oil of oregano). I then started taking a probiotic yeast called Saccharomyces boulardii.

Upon retesting, we found that we had eradicated the parasite and started to see signs that my gut bacteria were finally coming back into balance. Over this period, my bloating completely disappeared and, remarkably, my fatigue showed huge signs of improvement, which meant that I was able to return to work full-time, feeling healthier than I've ever felt before.

2. Replace

Note: if you are following an elimination diet for suspected food sensitivity or intolerance, this stage should come after the reintroduction-challenge phase (see p. 136).

This stage is all about including the types of foods that will nurture your health and nourish your body.

But first, let's talk about stomach acid. The role of stomach acid is to protect your body against invaders and digest food. As with anything, a delicate balance is needed (we call this 'the sweet spot') to ensure that you don't run into trouble.

It is commonly assumed that most cases of indigestion are related to high stomach acid, which is thought to cause gut issues like acid reflux and nausea. However, low stomach acid is even more common, and it can also lead to these symptoms, as well as other digestive and health-related difficulties. Low stomach acid can also drive bacterial overgrowth (SIBO) in the upper gut and worsen feelings of fatigue as a result.

Either scenario can make it difficult to break down food and absorb nutrients from our diets, which, as we know, is a real problem when we rely so heavily on specific nutrients to manufacture energy. Plus, digestion itself is energetically very demanding.

The baking soda test (opposite) will measure your stomach-acid levels to give you a rough idea of whether you are high or low on the spectrum:

THE BAKING SODA TEST

Do this test as soon as you wake up in the morning, before you have brushed your teeth or had anything to eat or drink:

- Dissolve ¼ teaspoon of bicarbonate of soda (baking soda) in ½ cup of filtered cold water.
- Drink the solution.
- Set a five-minute timer and record how long it takes you to burp.

If you have adequate amounts of stomach acid, you should burp within two to three minutes. If you burp immediately or before two minutes, it could be that you have high stomach acid. If it takes longer than three minutes, or you do not burp at all, it may be that you are not producing enough stomach acid. Perform on three consecutive days to get an average.

Optimise your stomach acid

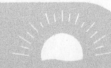

For low stomach acid:

- Try drinking apple cider vinegar before each meal. Start with 1 tablespoon and dilute in a glass of water; you should get a feeling of warmth in your stomach. If you don't get that sensation, increase the amount to 2 or 3 tablespoons (but stop if you feel a burning sensation).

- Eat bitter foods and herbs, which can support the secretion of stomach acid. Examples include dandelion greens, dill, bitter melon, burdock and chamomile.

- Consider taking a supplement called betaine HCL. However, I'd advise consulting a practitioner before supplementing, especially because you will need to rule out high stomach acid, too. (**Note:** betaine HCL is not recommended if you are pregnant, breastfeeding or have a history of gastritis or ulcers.)

- Chronic stress can lead to low stomach acid. You may also need to consider medications that may be lowering your stomach acid.

For high stomach acid:

- Incorporate marshmallow-root tea into your routine (loose leaf). Marshmallow root is a herb that can support and protect the gut from damage if stomach acid is raised and flowing back up into the oesophagus.

- Speak with a healthcare practitioner about taking deglycyrrhizinated liquorice for high stomach acid. (**Note:** check with a healthcare professional if you are pregnant or breastfeeding, or if you are taking any medication.)

- Working on stress is pivotal here, too, to lower stomach acid.

It's not just what you eat – it's how you eat!
When there is digestive disarray, it is easy to blame our diets. And while this is a factor, consideration should also be given to *how* we eat.

Some professionals argue that digestion begins in the mouth, when we chew our food (a process known as mastication). But the digestion process really begins just before this, when we start to engage with the *idea* of eating. Named the cephalic phase of digestion – when we tune in to our senses and look at food, think about it, smell it and begin to anticipate the process of eating it – this is the point at which we start to release salivary enzymes and stomach acid. In fact, approximately 20 per cent of our total stomach-acid secretion begins during the cephalic phase, before food has even entered our mouths.

So here are some guidelines on *how* to eat for optimal functioning of the digestive process:

- Banish distractions (no social media or TV) around eating times to enjoy the ritual of eating in its entirety.

- Chew your food fifteen to twenty times before swallowing to activate enzymes that aid food breakdown. Food should be around a liquid consistency before it is swallowed (remember, we do not have teeth in our stomachs).

- Practise mindfulness in the moment, savouring the flavours and textures of your food as you eat.

- Try putting your knife and fork down to pause between bites, to support your hunger hormones in receiving fullness signals; the longer you take to eat, the more likely you are to register your fullness without overeating and stay in tune with satiety signals.

- Don't force yourself to clear your plate. You don't need to feel uncomfortably full to leave the dinner table; your body is not a dustbin, after all.

The importance of digestive enzymes and bile

Digestive enzymes are proteins that speed up the chemical processes that break down food into smaller substances for the purposes of digestion. Our bodies produce certain enzymes naturally (in our pancreas and liver, for example), but many are delivered to us through what we eat.

I commonly see pancreatic insufficiency in clinical practice, which can result in nutritional deficiencies and yep, you guessed it, fatigue, which may warrant the use of digestive-enzyme supplements for a period. As always, work with a practitioner when it comes to supplementation.

Incorporate natural enzyme-rich foods into your diet such as:

- Papaya[S, H]
- Pineapple[S, H]
- Avocado[F, H]

- Kiwi[H]
- Ginger

You also need to think about bile (a greenish–yellow fluid produced by the liver and stored in the gallbladder). Bile contains bile salts, which help the body to digest fats and absorb fat-soluble vitamins (such as A, D, E and K). They also play a role in getting rid of toxins from the body. Bile and bile-salt deficiencies can contribute to digestive issues and nutritional deficiencies (particularly, A, D, E and K). If you suspect that you have a problem breaking down fats, you may need to consider supplementing with bile salts or a bile extract (see p. 178). Incidentally, drinking lemon juice in water can stimulate bile production in the liver, so it's a great thing to add to your morning routine.

Give your gut a break

The replace stage is all about supporting your gut and its inherent needs, which includes fuelling it with the right types of foods, but you also need to know when to give it some respite.

Time-restricted eating is a type of intermittent fasting that limits your eating window to a certain number of hours within a twenty-four-hour period. It can be useful for metabolic, immune and digestive health and is a lifestyle strategy to consider if you have CFS.

When I work with CFS clients, I often play around with the 16:8 and 14:10 approaches, which involve fasting for either sixteen or fourteen hours of the day and eating within an eight- or ten-hour window. This might involve eating your evening meal at 8pm and then not eating again until 12pm the next day, for example (16:8), or eating your first meal of the day at 9am and then not eating anything after 7pm (14:10). There are numerous benefits to be had from time-restricted eating:

- **Digestive clear-up** We have a housekeeping mechanism in our gut called the migrating motor complex (MMC). This is like an electrical wave of sweeping activity that clears out undigested food particles, debris and bacteria from the stomach and small intestine, reducing the likelihood of dysbiosis and bacteria ending up in places they wouldn't normally be (such as the small intestine). Fasting and spacing your meals out by around four hours helps this process and is a helpful tool to reboot the gut and support the activity of the microbiome.

- **Cellular clear-up** Fasting is a fantastic tool to manipulate our cells and the immune system for the better. Fasting upregulates a process called autophagy (this translates to 'self-eating', where the body can break down damaged and redundant cells, which is essential for the immune system to function optimally and thrive). Autophagy can also help to clear out autoantibodies, which underlie autoimmune processes, as well as breaking down dysfunctional mitochondria.

- **Blood-sugar regulation**: studies have shown favourable outcomes of time-restricting eating on blood-sugar regulation.

Limitations of time-restricted eating in CFS

- It may be problematic in the initial stages for those with HPA axis dysfunction who are prone to low blood sugar and food cravings.

- It may also be initially problematic for those with co-morbidities such as type-1 or type-2 diabetes if they are taking insulin injections or medications to lower blood sugar.

- It may exacerbate feelings of fatigue in some individuals.

These factors must always be weighed up and addressed when working with CFS, due to bio-individuality. Speak to a practitioner to see if this is something that might be right for your situation.

So what on earth do I eat?

Remember, it's not just about what you remove – what you *include* in your diet matters, too – hence the 'replace' phase.

GREEN LEAFY VEGETABLES

Green leafy vegetables are nutritional powerhouses filled with fibre, vitamins, minerals and phytonutrients (plant chemicals) that can support health, including vitamins A, C, K, calcium and potassium. When it comes to CFS, these leafy veg also deliver a bonanza of fatigue-fighting nutrients such as folate, magnesium and iron.

Try to include at least one cup of green leafy vegetables in your diet each day. Enjoy your greens with a small serving of extra virgin olive oil, since the fat content will aid the absorption of fat-soluble nutrients such as vitamins A and K. Examples include:

- Spinach[H, S]
- Swiss chard[S]
- Collard greens[S]
- Watercress[S]
- Romaine lettuce
- Chicory
- Napa cabbage (also known as Chinese leaf)*[S]
- Rocket*[S]
- Pak choi*[S]
- Kale*[S]
- Cauliflower*[F, S]
- Beet greens

* Also classed as cruciferous vegetables (see below).

CRUCIFEROUS VEGETABLES

These include:

- Rocket[S]
- Broccoli[S]
- Pak choi[S]
- Kale[S]

- Cauliflower[F, S]
- Radish[S]
- Brussels sprouts[F, S]
- Cabbage[S]
- Napa cabbage (also known as Chinese leaf)[S]
- Turnips[S]

These foods are rich in vitamins and minerals, as well as phyto-nutrients, such as glucosinolates – sulphur-containing compounds that the body digests and breaks down into many different compounds, including sulforaphane. Sulforaphane is known for its antioxidant and anti-inflammatory benefits. Studies have also shown that it can main-tain the health of the blood–brain barrier, which shows promise for those battling brain fog and neuroinflammation (inflammation in the brain).[8] It also helps the liver to excrete toxins and waste materials more easily out of the body.

However, there are also some potential drawbacks to consuming cruciferous vegetables, which you should consider if you have CFS. The first is their goitrogen content, which can block the function of the thyroid, and, in extreme cases, lead to the development of a goitre (a swelling in the neck resulting from an enlargement of the thyroid gland).

Did you know?

Broccoli sprouts (essentially, the baby version of broccoli) are a microgreen containing 100 times more sulforaphane than a fully grown broccoli head. Generally consumed raw, broccoli sprouts retain more nutritional value – so if you don't have a sulphur intolerance and have ruled out iodine deficiency, add them to your soups, salads and stews for a nutrient-packed hit.

If you have discovered that you have an iodine deficiency (which may result in thyroid insufficiency and lie at the heart of your CFS symp-toms), I recommend that you are mindful about how many cruciferous vegetables you consume raw and aim for no more than half a cup each day. You can always cook or ferment cruciferous vegetables, though, which helps to break down some of their goitrogen content.

The second concern is that if sulphur intolerance is an issue for you, you may need to work on reducing these foods initially, until you have supported your body's ability to better metabolise sulphur-rich foods once again.

B-VITAMIN FOODS

This family of eight vitamins is essential when battling CFS to ensure that you provide your body with everything it needs to manufacture energy at a cellular level, and that the methylation process is working efficiently. B vitamin stores need to be replenished through the diet each day, especially when we are chronically stressed because they can become depleted during such metabolically demanding times.

Foods that are naturally rich in B-vitamins include:

- Wholegrains such as brown rice[S] and oats[S]
- Eggs[S]
- Liver[S], chicken[S], turkey[S], mackerel[H], salmon
- Spinach[H, S] and kale[S]
- Avocados[F, H]
- Asparagus[F, S]
- Chickpeas[F, S, H], kidney beans[F, S, H], black beans[F, S, H], green peas[F, S, H]
- Sunflower seeds

Note: vitamin B12 is found exclusively in animal products; therefore vegans will need to take a B12 supplement (see p. 178). Also, some CFS patients have genetic variants (SNPs) that impair their ability to methylate. Methylated B vitamin supplements can be helpful in these individuals (see p. 178).

OMEGA-3 FATTY ACIDS

An essential fat is a type of fat that must be consumed in the diet for the body to stay healthy. Omega-3 fatty acids are essential fats that play numerous roles in keeping our bodies running in tip-top condition. These structural fats are vital in forming our cellular membranes and are found abundantly in the brain. In fact, 60 per cent of the brain is made up of fat, which is why essential fats such as omega-3 are so crucial to its health and smooth functioning.

If you think of your brain as a house made up of bricks, then one in every three of these bricks is made up of omega-3 fatty acids, which form its outer membrane. Not only do they help to form the structure of our brains, they can also play a role in cellular signalling and neural firing. This is an essential part of maintaining and promoting health, particularly cognition, which is why omega-3s can be highly supportive for those with brain fog. Research has also shown that omega-3 fats are very good at fighting chronic inflammation, a process that, as we know, underlies many chronic diseases.[9]

Omega-3s are found in oily fish such as salmon, mackerel, anchovies, sardines and herring (I use the acronym SMASH to help remember these). Unfortunately, however, the level of omega-3s in our oily fish is starting to decline, particularly when it comes to farmed sources, meaning that more and more of us are becoming depleted in these key essential fats and need to consider supplementation.

Omega-3s can also be found in plant-based foods such as flax, hemp, chia seeds and walnuts. But vegans or vegetarians (or those who aren't fans of oily fish) may still want to consider supplementing (see p. 178).

Aim for at least two 140g portions of oily fish per week (try including wild-caught if you are having salmon), or for vegans/vegetarians opt for an algae-based supplement containing a minimum of 500mg EPA and DHA combined.

FABULOUS FIBRE

Every time you eat, you are not just feeding yourself but also the trillions of microbes that live within your gut.

When the food we eat hits the large intestine, beneficial bacteria colonies in the gut get to work on the dietary fibre. They 'gobble up' what we ourselves cannot digest and produce substances called short-chain fatty acids (SCFAs). These act as a fuel source for the cells that line the colon and can dampen down inflammation, helping to maintain the integrity of the gut lining. Therefore, a healthy level of SCFAs is supportive of overall health and, of course, in dealing with CFS. SCFAs are known as 'postbiotics' and are being investigated for their health benefits.

Close to 100 different types of fibre have been identified, which is why a diverse diet is key to gaining a cocktail of different fibres for gut health. It's recommended that adults consume 30g fibre a day, although most of us only achieve around 18g daily. The more plants that you can add to your plate, the easier it will be to hit your daily fibre quota. Add nuts and seeds to your breakfast bowl, snack on raw carrot sticks dipped in houmous and keep the skins on your vegetables to up your fibre intake. If you don't currently consume lots of fibre, always go low and slow – introducing small amounts slowly over time – otherwise your gut bacteria will have a field day and produce a lot of gas!

PREBIOTICS

Prebiotics are a food source for the beneficial bacteria that reside within the gut, promoting their growth and increasing their number (think fertiliser for your inner gut garden).

A diverse ecosystem of friendly gut bacteria is favourable for overall health and can support those with dysbiosis, as well as tackling the various other chronic stressors that are thought to underlie CFS.

Only a subset of dietary fibres qualify as prebiotic. What's more, prebiotics can also come from non-fibre substances, such as polyphenols (chemicals found in plants that have potent antioxidant properties). Plus, they can also be taken in supplement form.

Prebiotics from the fibre camp include inulin, pectin, beta-glucans, resistant starch, partially hydrolysed guar gum, fructo-oligosaccharides (FOS), galacto-oligosaccharides (GOS) and xylo-oligosaccharides (XOS). They are found in chicory, Jerusalem artichokes[F, S], asparagus (raw)[S], banana (the greener and less ripe, the higher the prebiotic content)[H], oats[S], apples[F], garlic[F, S], leeks[F, S] and onions[F, S].

Prebiotics from the polyphenol camp include flavonoids, phenolic acids, resveratrol, lignans. They are found in apples[F], onions[F, S], grapes[F], citrus fruits[H], wholegrains[S], raspberries[F] and flax seeds.

There is no official recommended guideline for prebiotic intake, but a good starting point is approximately 5g per day.

Note: prebiotic fibres are most notably associated with an increase in SCFAs (see the previous page).

FERMENTED FOODS

Fermentation is a process that involves bacteria and yeasts breaking down sugars in certain foods to enhance preservation, as well as to increase the number of beneficial microorganisms in those foods.

Fermented foods are often used interchangeably with the term 'probiotic'. A probiotic refers to live microorganisms that, when consumed in adequate quantities, confer a health benefit on the person taking them. However, not all fermented foods qualify as probiotic (beer, for example), and not all probiotics take the form of fermented foods (they can also come in supplement form – see p. 178). That said, it is still possible for some foods to be considered both probiotic and fermented – for example:

- Sauerkraut[F, H, S] – made from shredded, fermented cabbage and salt
- Kimchi[F, H] – sauerkraut's Korean friend; a spicy fermented cabbage
- Miso[H, S] – a paste that is fermented and made from soy (or sometimes grains)
- Bio yoghurt[F, H, S] – while most yoghurt is traditionally fermented with bacteria (classed as 'live'), bio yoghurt has additional cultures of friendly bacteria added to it after fermentation, resulting in higher numbers of good bacteria (you can always check the label to see if it contains 'live cultures')
- Kefir[F, H, S] – a fermented milk drink, made using 'kefir grains', which are gelatinous beads of yeast and bacteria
- Kombucha[F, H] – a fermented, effervescent black or green tea drink

The process of fermentation helps to break down nutrients (and even antinutrients, more of which on pp. 171–172) in food, making them easier to digest than their unfermented counterparts. Try to consume fermented foods daily – say, 1–2 tablespoons of sauerkraut or kimchi alongside your morning eggs or with a mackerel salad.

Do be mindful if you have FODMAP, histamine or sulphur issues, however, as fermented foods can be a huge culprit for triggering symptoms if you are prone to reactions. Be mindful with fermented foods if you have SIBO, too, because you don't want to add to the load if there is already a bacterial overgrowth in the upper gut.

However, consuming healthy fermented foods in the diet can be very helpful if you have dysbiosis in the gut due to a lack of beneficial bacteria or even a poor diversity of gut microbes.

Top tip: always opt for unpasteurised (i.e. non-heated) fermented foods, which help to keep the bacteria intact to confer their health benefits.

ANTI-INFLAMMATORY SPICES

When we think about fighting inflammation, two well-known wonder spices come to mind: ginger and turmeric.

Ginger contains gingerols, which have been shown in studies to have antioxidants and inflammation-fighting properties[10], as does curcumin, the active compound in turmeric.[11] Incorporate these spices into your cooking routine. Try grating a generous wedge of ginger into your evening stir-fry or sprinkling a dash of turmeric powder into a home-made Thai curry.

IODINE IN THE DIET

Iodine is crucial for the thyroid gland since it is required to make thyroid hormones. And it also supports the production of stomach acid.

The body does not naturally make iodine, so we need to get this key nutrient through our diets. It is found in the following foods:

- Seaweed (for example, kelp, dulse, nori, furikake)
- Eggs[S]
- Oysters[H]
- Fish (haddock, cod and plaice)[S]
- Yoghurt and other dairy products[H, S, F]
- Iodised salt (most salt in the UK is non-iodised)

The official recommended daily intake of iodine for the average adult is 140mcg.

Iodine is a 'Goldilocks' nutrient, which means that you need just the right amount of it in the body, depending on what your thyroid function looks like.

It is best to avoid heavy consumption of very concentrated sources of iodine, such as seaweed (I would advise against consuming this more than twice per week). And avoid artificially iodised salt, too. Focus instead on obtaining iodine from other dietary sources, as listed previously.

Those particularly at risk of iodine deficiency include vegans and vegetarians who do not consume many iodine-rich foods. But always seek the advice of a healthcare professional; you must be very careful about how much iodine you take as it can worsen thyroid problems.

SELENIUM

Selenium is a trace mineral and antioxidant that is supportive for the immune system. It is also crucial for the creation of thyroid hormones. This is why a selenium deficiency could explain symptoms of CFS if thyroid insufficiency is at the heart of it.

Selenium is found in the following:

- Brazil nuts[S]
- Sardines[H], halibut[S], oysters[H], crab[S, H], salmon[S]
- Beef[S], turkey[S], chicken[S]
- Eggs[S]
- Brown rice[S]
- Oats[S]
- Sunflower seeds
- Mushrooms[F, H]

The amount of selenium in plant-based foods can vary, depending on the selenium content of the soil in which they are grown. Because it is scarce in UK soils, vegetarians and vegans may run the risk of a selenium deficiency.

Just like iodine, selenium is a nutrient that needs to be finely balanced, as toxicity is possible if you overdo it. Eat two to three Brazil nuts per day (or consume the other sources listed above) to obtain enough selenium to prevent deficiency.

You may consider selenium supplementation if there is a deficiency or if it is a struggle to obtain and absorb what you need in the diet. Avoid taking more than 400mcg a day and, if in doubt, get your levels checked and go from there.

Ⅱ

IRON-RICH FOODS

Iron is a mineral that the body uses to make haemoglobin, a protein in red blood cells that carries oxygen from the lungs to different parts of the body. A lack of iron can lead to iron-deficiency anaemia, and those who are especially vulnerable include vegans, vegetarians and those with malabsorption issues, as well as women who experience heavy blood loss through menstruation.

Not only is iron critical for oxygenation of bodily tissues, it is also a big deal for thyroid hormone conversion, making it a key factor in the fight against fatigue.

There are two forms of iron in the diet: haem and non-haem. Haem iron is found in animal proteins (such as beef, poultry, oysters and sardines) and is more absorbable than non-haem iron, which is found in plant-based sources, such as beans, tofu, apricots, collard greens, kale, nuts, seeds and lentils.

If you pair non-haem iron with vitamin C, you will increase the absorption rate; so next time you sit down to eat a beany chili or a kale salad, squeeze over some lime or lemon juice (rich in vitamin C) to maximise iron absorption. You should also avoid tea or coffee with your iron food sources, because the tannin content can hinder iron absorption.

If you are vegan or vegetarian, you will need to consume almost double the recommended intake of iron to prevent deficiency.

It's a good idea to get your iron levels checked if you think you may be deficient (see p. 114) – that way you can focus on the amount of iron to include in your diet and go from there.

Too much iron (known as iron overload) is also a possibility and can result in toxicity. This can happen if you overdose on iron supplements, take high-dose iron supplements for a long time or if you suffer from a chronic iron-overload condition (such as haemochromatosis – a genetic disorder where the gut absorbs dangerously high amounts of iron from the diet). Unless you have such a disorder, you don't really need to worry about getting too much iron in the diet, but you should be mindful about supplementation (see p. 177).

If you need to increase your iron intake, focus on the following foods:

- Liver[S], beef[S] and chicken[S]
- Sardines[H] and oysters[H]
- Pumpkin seeds
- Quinoa[S]
- Chickpeas[F, S, H]
- Lentils[F, S, H]
- Blackstrap molasses[F, S] (1 tablespoon is about a quarter of your daily iron requirement, but be mindful of the sugar content and try to have it with a source of protein)
- Spinach[H, S]
- Broccoli [S]

Mix it up!
I always tell my clients 'diversity is the spice of life', and this is certainly true when it comes to achieving a healthy, balanced diet.

A healthy diet relies on a cocktail of plant-based chemicals and a variety of different vitamins, minerals and fibres. So if, say, you are eating blueberries every day with your porridge, you will be taking in fibre and polyphenols to feed some species of friendly gut bacteria, but you'll also be denying other beneficial communities of gut microbes the types of fibres and plant chemicals that they thrive off, which are found in buckwheat, flax, blackberries, raspberries or cherries, for example.

Try to purchase at least two new plant-based foods at the supermarket every week to ensure that you rotate your diet and always incorporate something plant-based and different. This will also help when it comes to testing your tolerance profiles, if food sensitivity and intolerance have been underlying issues in your battle with CFS (you can then start to experiment and broaden your diet out once again). Overall, the aim of the game is to have an inclusive, diverse and embracing approach towards food that doesn't trigger symptoms.

Balance your plate
If your diet includes animal products, a balanced plate will typically look like this:

- 1 or 2 palm-sized servings of lean protein, such as chicken, fish, turkey, prawns (but do be mindful of animal protein if there is a sulphur intolerance)
- 1 fistful of complex carbohydrates, such as sweet potato, lentils, brown rice, quinoa
- 2 fistfuls of non-starchy vegetables, such as kale, rocket, courgette, broccoli, bell pepper, tomato, carrot, cauliflower
- 1–2 tablespoon-sized servings of healthy fats, such as sunflower seeds, walnuts, avocado, extra virgin olive oil

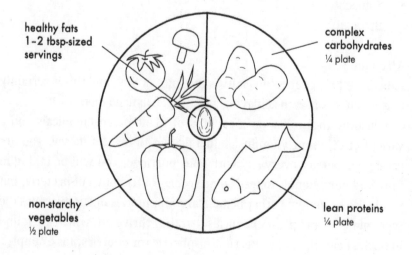

healthy fats
1–2 tbsp-sized
servings

complex
carbohydrates
¼ plate

non-starchy
vegetables
½ plate

lean proteins
¼ plate

If you follow a vegan diet, your sources of protein will instead be bound to complex carbohydrates including tempeh, edamame, quinoa, lentils, or to sources of healthy fats, including chia seeds, peanuts and hemp seeds. Your plant protein should make up half of your plate, while the other half should be non-starchy vegetables. Make sure you incorporate a combination of complex carbs and fats to ensure you don't miss out on any macronutrients (namely, protein, carbohydrates and fat – required in larger amounts in the diet to stay healthy).

For vegetarians, sources of protein will be bound to animal sources, such as eggs and dairy, and also to plant-based sources, such as wholegrains, legumes, nuts and seeds. Your plate should be half non-starchy vegetables, a quarter animal proteins (eggs, for example) and a quarter plant proteins (nuts, seeds, legumes, wholegrains), with around 1–2 tablespoons of healthy fats.

Top tip: eat thirty plants a week. Keep this number in mind as a weekly target when incorporating whole foods into your diet. This includes fruits, vegetables, nuts, seeds, wholegrains and legumes. Herbs and spices are also great, each being worth a quarter of a point towards your plant intake. However, always be realistic about what you can really incorporate into your routine with CFS and don't beat yourself up if you don't quite hit this quota.

Make life easy for yourself!

Enlist help, plan, batch cook and freeze your food. Always be realistic about how much you can cook for yourself with the energy you have and be prepared to make things easier. Remember that a diet that is too stressful will only hinder not help your situation.

There are some great healthy-meal-delivery companies that offer recipe kits and quick meals to save you time and energy. Some great examples include Mindful Chef and The Detox Kitchen, and both deliver straight to your door.

Low carb, not no carb

All too often, I see people cutting out carbohydrates, which are essential for energy production and supporting a balanced mood. While you can certainly benefit from reducing the sugars and starches in your diet if you have CFS, it doesn't mean you need to avoid carbs completely. Think low carb, not no carb, and focus on the right *types* of carbohydrate, which include complex carbohydrates found in sweet potatoes, squash, brown rice, quinoa and lentils, for instance.

Increase bioavailability

Bioavailability refers to how well nutrients are absorbed within the body and, of course, with CFS you want to make sure that you maximise this to get the best possible nutritional benefit.

To increase bioavailability, be mindful of antinutrients (compounds in food that can irritate the gut lining, hinder digestion and inhibit the absorption of nutrients).

The highest concentrations of antinutrients are found in legumes, nuts, grains and seeds, as well as in spinach, tea and coffee. Luckily, however, we can deactivate and reduce amounts of these compounds to lessen their impact. This involves certain food preparation methods, as follows:

- **Soaking:** soaking grains, nuts, seeds and legumes in water (sometimes overnight) and draining them before preparation is a way to deactivate the antinutrients contained within.

- **Sprouting:** also known as germination, sprouting involves soaking grains, nuts, seeds and legumes in water for several hours, and then repeatedly rinsing them, until they begin to sprout or develop a tail-like protrusion.

- **Fermenting:** fermentation involves submerging a food in brine in a sealed container and leaving it over time (commonly a few days to a few weeks, depending on the food) to deactivate the antinutrients, while also increasing beneficial bacteria.

- **Steaming:** try to steam your vegetables instead of boiling them; this will not only reduce the antinutrient content, but also helps to retain most nutrients, which can otherwise leach into the water in other cooking processes, such as boiling.

Top tip: avoid consuming too many raw foods that have not been prepared appropriately (soaked, steamed or fermented), so that you do not overload on antinutrients, which could interfere with your gut and nutritional status.

Hydrate, hydrate, hydrate
The human body is made up of 60 per cent water, so it is no surprise that drinking more H_2O is one of my top recommendations in clinic for supporting health.

Water helps our cells to function efficiently and absorb nutrients, while promoting digestion, supporting cognition and detoxification (including the excretion of toxins). Every chemical reaction that takes place in the brain requires water, especially energy production. The brain is *very* sensitive to dehydration, and we can feel lacklustre if we don't drink enough of it day to day.

How much water you require depends on your age, sex, physical activity levels and overall health status. As a guideline, you should aim to drink 1.5–2 litres daily. So instead of drinking sugar-sweetened beverages (this includes fruit juices, too), buy yourself a sustainable and reusable water bottle and get drinking! Flavour with fruits and herbs, such as cucumbers, lemon, lime, berries or a sprig of fresh rosemary or mint.

Top tip: if your urine is bright yellow, you may be dehydrated. Aim for a champagne or straw colour for optimum hydration.

3. Reinoculate

It is now time to think about addressing any imbalances in your gut by reinoculating with some beneficial bacteria supplements (probiotics).

Because CFS exists as a syndrome of symptoms, it is hard to nail down one specific probiotic species or product that works to improve health outcomes for all patients. In fact, many probiotic research trials only look at potential benefits on one specific symptom (such as fatigue) or a physiological process (say, inflammation).

This means that the evidence around taking probiotics for CFS is mixed. I am also a firm believer in using a personalised regime of probiotics in CFS to balance the microbiome and support dysbiosis of the gut, and I tend to see really great results with this in terms of fatigue, digestive and neurological health in my CFS clients. Interestingly, studies are also now looking into probiotic therapy for those hospitalised with COVID-19, aimed at preventing chronic fatigue after discharge.[12]

On the flip side, sometimes taking a probiotic can run us into problems. In the past, I have seen stool test results skewed towards an overgrowth of friendly bacteria, a form of dysbiosis, which means that taking a probiotic may not be very wise in these cases. It's about finding a balance of friendly microbes and avoiding too much of a good thing.

Some key genera of bacteria that may be of relevance in CFS include Bifidobacteria, Faecalibacterium and Lactobacillus, and the species and strains within these camps undergoing research in the field of CFS.

Here are some points to consider when purchasing a probiotic:

- One of the first things to understand about probiotics is that they are not all created equal. Products can differ in the strain, strength and delivery system of the probiotic cultures.

- Another important thing to consider is whether the product you are purchasing has been specially formulated to protect the bacteria when they reach the acid in the stomach, so that the probiotics remain intact in transit to the colon (this applies regardless of whether the supplement is in capsule or liquid form).

- The quantity of bacteria in a probiotic does not always equal quality, so a product that claims it delivers 20 billion CFUs (colony-forming units) versus one that contains 10 billion may not necessarily be better.

- A stool test may help you to navigate your probiotic choices.

Note: as ever, always consult a healthcare professional before considering supplementation, especially if you are pregnant or taking any medication.

4. Repair

This stage of the 5R plan involves nurturing the gut lining, which, as we've covered, can become 'leaky' (see p. 76) due to various dietary and lifestyle factors – sugar, food sensitivities (gluten, for example), alcohol, medications, infections – leading to chronic inflammation.

We covered how food sensitivities play a role in intestinal permeability, and how when these are present and you simply remove a particular food, it may take away the irritant, but it does not necessarily repair the terrain. A saying I find useful here is, 'If a hammer breaks a window, removing the hammer does not repair the window.'

To achieve a healthy mucosal barrier that keeps tight junctions intact, the gut requires proteins in the form of:

- glutamine
- glycine
- collagen
- gelatine.

If you are willing to consume animal products, then bone broth (from

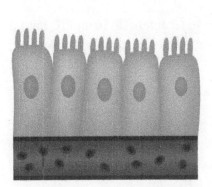
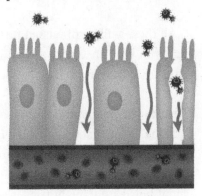

Normal tight junction   **Leaky and inflamed**

beef or chicken) is a fantastic source of gut-nurturing nutrients (it contains all the proteins listed above). However, if you follow a plant-based or vegetarian diet, you might want to consider a supplement. Glutamine, for example, is a real hero that has been shown in studies to be excellent at repairing a leaky gut.[13] (**Note:** if you have histamine or sulphur intolerance, opt for a glutamine supplement instead of consuming bone broth.)

As you move forwards in your recovery, you will start to see your food sensitivities improving and that you can handle a much wider variety of foods once again. This is a positive indication that your health is on the up, and that gut integrity is being restored. The fewer sensitivities you have, the more robust your gut lining will be, and this is proof positive that recovery is taking place.

5. Rebalance

This step of the plan is largely about addressing lifestyle habits that have an enormous influence on your health, particularly fatigue. During this phase, you will want to consider:

- activity management (including pacing and grading)

- improving sleep
- stress management (SNS support)
- eliminating environmental toxins (including moulds, pesticides, heavy metals) and supporting detoxification
- improving mental resilience and wellbeing.

All these will be discussed further in Chapters 15, 16 and 17, but for now the rebalance phase is all about finding a suitable diet for your long-term health and happiness.

Healing your relationship with food

It's safe to say that when food triggers are contributing to your chronic illness, your relationship with food can go awry. That's why focusing on it is important, so that you do not become overly phobic or worried about how eating might trigger your CFS symptoms.

We often associate food with our symptoms, which can indeed be a reality. However, it is equally important to recognise that food is just *one* part of the jigsaw puzzle, and not the whole story. Remember that illnesses like CFS are incredibly complex and multifaceted, which means that you need to find the right diet that works for you, exploring this area using a personalised approach – because, after all, we are each biochemically unique.

What resonated with me in my own recovery from CFS was not just battling the chronic symptoms daily, but the times when I felt like I missed out on socialising, not being able to eat various things and join in the party like everybody else. At one stage, I was following an auto-immune protocol (AIP, also known as the autoimmune paleo diet), and I felt endlessly paranoid about food at restaurants being 'contaminated' with trace amounts of things I was not permitted, afraid that this would cause another crash or symptom exacerbation. I was so consumed by the fear of trigger foods that I was not only miserable about my health, but even more miserable about feeling so restricted with my diet.

Yet all the while, stress and anxiety around food were compounding my health problem. My nervous system was chronically activated in fight-or-flight mode, with cortisol and adrenaline being triggered no end.

Having since adopted a more balanced approach towards eating and recovering my health, I have come to understand the importance of being mindful of how recovery diets can affect the mindset. In practice, this means that while viewing recovery from CFS through the lens of functional medicine, we must also apply a slice of common sense and not allow thoughts about food to become intrusive. Often, people experience what's known as a 'nocebo effect' – where negative expectations around eating a particular food elicit a negative response to it. So we need to remember at all times that food is essential – and that goes for the soul, as well as the body.

What's the score on supplements?

When it comes to supplementation, it really depends on identifying the root cause of your concerns and addressing the identified chronic stressors from there. This will mean factoring in your main presenting symptoms, lifestyle, budget, drug interactions, life stage and co-morbidities. No one supplement will be the sole answer to your recovery prayers; however, they can be pivotal in providing support along the way.

It's also important to mention that you should not use supplements to compensate for a bad diet – it's always best to make the nutritional changes outlined earlier in this chapter before you even consider supplementation.

Note: a lot of my CFS clients are very sensitive to supplements and can react badly to them if they are not careful. That's why the choice of supplement and dosages must be considered to avoid any exacerbation of symptoms. As always, do consult a healthcare professional when considering supplementation, especially if you are pregnant or taking medication.

The following nutrients might be considered for supplementation.

Why supplement?

We would consider supplementing in CFS in order to:

- correct a nutritional deficiency or to address a higher functional need for a particular nutrient (due to an organic acid test result, for example)
- support the organs involved in eliminating toxins (particularly if there is toxic overload)
- support the mitochondria
- fight oxidative stress
- reduce chronic inflammation
- support the adrenals and the stress response
- support the thyroid
- support the gut (especially if there is dysbiosis and leaky gut)
- help to tackle an infection (whether acute or chronic).

However, once again, these should *only and always* be taken in consultation with a healthcare professional:

- Magnesium
- CoQ10
- Carnitine
- Nicotinamide riboside
- Probiotics
- Glutathione
- N-acetyl-cysteine (NAC)
- Alpha-lipoic acid (ALA)
- Chromium
- Digestive enzymes
- B vitamins (including methylated B vitamins)
- D-ribose
- Chlorella
- Vitamin C
- Vitamin D
- Omega-3 fatty acids (EPA and DHA)
- Anti-microbials
- L-glutamine
- Bile salts
- Adaptogens
- Molybdenum
- Selenium
- Iodine
- Iron

- Zinc
- Peppermint oil
- Quercetin
- DAO (diamine oxidase)
- Curcumin

- Phosphatidylcholine (PC)
- Milk thistle
- Cistus incanus
- Colostrum
- Phosphatidylserine

WHAT ABOUT MULTIVITAMINS?

On occasion, multivitamins can be useful as a stopgap approach; but in CFS, there is often a much higher demand for more targeted support in certain areas, which multivitamins may struggle to address.

SUPPORTIVE SUPPLEMENTATION

A question I am often asked is: can you overdo it? And the reality is that taking too many supplements at once can become a real issue, as they start to compete for absorption in the body. Also, always opt for the better-absorbed forms (powders and liquids are great because they are rapidly taken up by the digestive system, which is useful if there are issues with breaking capsules down in the gut).

Top tip #1: watch out for supplement companies that use a variety of cheap binders and fillers and low-quality nutrients. Follow recommendations from a trusted practitioner if you are unsure. You want the best-quality nutrients with zero junk fillers, additives and binders.

Top tip #2: going low and slow is my motto. Due to sensitivities, it might be helpful to try introducing new supplements one at a time, to see whether they agree with you or not.

CHAPTER 14

Nutrition II - Recipes for Recovery

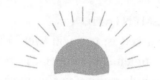

Let food be thy medicine, and medicine be thy food.
Hippocrates, Greek physician

You will likely find your own niche and ways of eating that suit your individual tolerance profile, so I'm not going to give you a plan to tell you exactly how to eat. With the recipes in this chapter, however, I have removed the low-hanging fruit – namely, gluten and dairy, two of the most common food sensitivities (plus some of the dishes are AIP-friendly, too).

Most of the recipes here serve one to four people, so if you do have extra servings, you can store or freeze them for another day, which always comes in handy if you are going through a crash. Some dishes can be prepared fresh or prepared in batches and refrigerated, so you can reheat them.

Note: check out www.ardere.com/recipes for further inspiration and photographs of many of these recipes.

Breakfast

Coconut and Flax Turmeric 'Porridge' with Stewed Apple

A grain-free porridge sensation, this one's quick to prepare and packs a wealth of fibre, including pectin, a prebiotic found in the stewed apple.

Serves: 1
Total time: 10 minutes

1 apple, cored and cubed
1 tsp cinnamon powder (plus extra for the stewed apple)
3 tbsp desiccated coconut
3 tbsp flaxseed powder
80ml almond milk
1 tsp ground turmeric

1 tsp honey (or maple syrup if you are vegan)
1 tbsp coconut yoghurt (optional)
20g walnuts, chopped or broken into pieces

1. Simmer the apple pieces in a saucepan over a medium heat with a splash of water. Add a sprinkle of cinnamon and stir for 10 minutes, until softened and sweet, adding more water if required.

2. Meanwhile, mix together the remaining ingredients in a bowl (apart from the walnuts and coconut yoghurt, if using).

3. Serve the apple and walnuts on top of your 'porridge' with the coconut yoghurt, if using.

Avocado Egg Boats

A fuss-free and fast breakfast that's high in healthy monounsaturated fats and protein and oozing with flavour. Need I say more?

Serves: 1
Total time: 25 minutes

1 large avocado, halved and
 stone removed
2 medium eggs
½ tsp chilli flakes

Salt and pepper
1 tbsp coriander leaves
 (optional)
Handful of rocket (optional)

1. Preheat the oven to 225°C.

2. Scoop out some of the flesh of each avocado half with a spoon until the shells are large enough to fit your eggs. You can save the extra avocado to serve on the side or enjoy as a snack.

3. Crack an egg into each avocado half and sprinkle with some chilli flakes and salt and pepper.

4. Bake in the oven for 20 minutes, or until the white is set and the yolk is still slightly runny.

5. Sprinkle some coriander leaves over the top and serve with rocket on the side, if using.

Kiwi and Spinach Chia Pudding

Not your average pudding, this is a source of green goodness and is also high in protein. Kiwi is fantastic for digestive regularity, while spinach provides a cocktail of fatigue-fighting nutrients from folate and iron to vitamin C and magnesium, to name just a few.

Serves: 2
Total time: 5 minutes

500ml coconut milk　　　　　**85g chia seeds**
Handful of spinach　　　　　**4 kiwis, peeled and diced**

1. Add the coconut milk and spinach to a blender and blitz, until combined and smooth.

2. Pour the mixture into a large bowl and add the chia seeds. Stir for 3 minutes, until the chia seeds start to swell and thicken.

3. Divide the kiwi evenly between two glass tumblers and spoon the chia-seed/spinach mixture over the top.

   Tip: best made and refrigerated the night before to be enjoyed chilled the next day.

Spicy Scrambled Eggs with Heirloom Tomato Salad, Smoked Salmon and Kimchi

A perfectly balanced plate with a touch of spice, this one will keep you going until lunchtime. Slow-cooked eggs provide a rich and creamy texture without the need for dairy products, while the smoked salmon is a rich source of omega-3 fats to support brain function. Kimchi finishes it all off by adding some probiotic goodness.

Serves: 1
Total time: 15 minutes

3 eggs
½ tsp chilli flakes
Pinch of salt and pepper
1 tsp olive oil
50g (2 slices) smoked salmon
150g heirloom tomatoes,

chopped into half-moons
1 heaped tbsp kimchi
Handful of rocket
1 tbsp chives, finely chopped
1 tbsp pine nuts

1. Crack the eggs into a bowl along with the chilli flakes and salt and pepper and whisk until smooth.

2. Heat the olive oil in a frying pan over a low–medium heat.

3. Add the egg mixture to the pan and cook for 8–10 minutes. Turn up the temperature very slightly towards the end if the eggs still need to firm up, then gently fold them into the middle of the pan, bit by bit, using a spoon.

4. Arrange the smoked salmon, tomatoes, kimchi and rocket on a plate.

5. Once the eggs are cooked to your desired consistency, serve alongside the salad with the chives and pine nuts sprinkled over the top.

Buckwheat Bircher Muesli with Grated Carrot and Pear

Buckwheat is a pseudograin that's high in a type of prebiotic fibre called resistant starch, which can feed your friendly gut bacteria. Paired with antioxidant-rich carrot and pear, this dish sets you up for a nourishing start to the day.

Serves: 1
Total time: 5 minutes

80g buckwheat flakes
175ml almond milk
1 carrot, peeled and grated

1 pear, cored and grated
1 tbsp chia seeds
25g sultanas (optional)

1. Mix all the ingredients together in a small bowl or glass tumbler.

2. Enjoy straight away or refrigerate overnight to allow the buckwheat to soak up the moisture from the almond milk. In the morning, remove from the fridge, adding a little more almond milk if needed.

Nutty Vanilla and Cinnamon Breakfast Parfaits

An indulgent choice for when you're craving something a little sweeter, this recipe is packed with healthy fats and protein, combined with some delicious spices and vanilla. Breakfast and dessert rolled into one!

Serves: 3
Total time: 30 minutes

45g flaked almonds
30g coconut flakes
1 tbsp coconut oil, melted
2 tsp ground cinnamon
½ tsp ground ginger
¼ tsp ground cardamom
50g pistachio nuts
15g Brazil nuts

15g hazelnuts
2 Medjool dates, pitted and chopped
1 tsp vanilla powder
25g ground flaxseed
20g desiccated coconut
250g coconut yoghurt

1. Preheat the oven to 150°C and line a baking tray with baking parchment.

2. In a bowl, mix the flaked almonds and coconut flakes with the coconut oil, 1 teaspoon of the cinnamon and the ginger and ground cardamom. Transfer to the baking tray and bake in the oven for 15 minutes.

3. Meanwhile, place all the remaining nuts, the Medjool dates, vanilla powder, flaxseed, desiccated coconut and the remaining cinnamon in a food processor. Pulse very briefly, so that it breaks down into smaller chunks but is not too fine.

4. Assemble your parfaits in three glass tumblers, starting with 2 tablespoons of coconut yoghurt in the base, followed by 3 tablespoons of the nutty flaxseed layer, and then a layer of 2 tablespoons of the flaked almonds and coconut. Repeat to create another layer in each glass.

Quinoa Porridge with Toasted Almond and Berry Sprinkle

A complete source of protein, quinoa is a pseudograin that makes for an excellent porridge base. Here, it's paired with antioxidant-rich berries to help in the fight against oxidative stress.

Serves: 1
Total time: 10 minutes

45g quinoa flakes
250ml coconut milk
1 heaped tbsp flaked almonds
Handful of blueberries

Handful of raspberries
½ tbsp honey, to serve (or maple syrup, if vegan)

1. Add the quinoa flakes to a small saucepan and then pour in the coconut milk.

2. Place over a medium heat for 3 minutes, until the porridge starts to thicken. Keep stirring and alter the temperature as needed, depending on how thick the porridge starts to get (you can always add more milk if you prefer a thinner consistency). Remove from the heat once cooked and pour into a breakfast bowl.

3. Meanwhile, toast the flaked almonds for 3–4 minutes in a pan over a medium heat. Keep a close eye on them, as they can burn very easily.

4. Sprinkle the blueberries and raspberries over the porridge and serve with the honey or maple syrup, as well as the toasted almond flakes.

Passion Fruit and Pomegranate Quick-Serve Yoghurt

Ready in just two minutes, this is the perfect breakfast to revive and refresh you when you're feeling time-poor and tired in the morning. Coconut yoghurt makes a great dairy-free alternative to regular yoghurt and combines well with vitamin-C-rich passion fruit and pomegranate.

Serves: 1
Total time: 2 minutes
Without the hemp seeds, this is AIP-friendly

150g natural coconut yoghurt
½ passion fruit
1 tbsp pomegranate seeds

1–2 tbsp shelled hemp seeds
(optional)

1. Smooth out the yoghurt into the base of a breakfast bowl.

2. Spoon the passion fruit into the yoghurt, stirring it through, until the yoghurt has turned an appetising orange colour, then stir through the pomegranate and hemp seeds (if using) and serve.

Leafy-Green Shakshuka
. . . .

A wonderful savoury egg sensation. The word 'shakshuka' translates to 'a mix-up', and that's exactly what this dish is: a mix-up of some of my favourite ingredients – leafy greens – packed full of fatigue-fighting nutrients, including iron, magnesium and folate.

Serves: 3
Total time: 20 minutes

1 tsp olive oil
3 shallots, finely sliced
1 green pepper, finely sliced
1 courgette, diced
100g green peas
1 tsp cumin
½ tsp oregano
Pinch of chilli flakes

Pinch of salt and pepper
Large handful of spinach
100g cavolo nero, trimmed to
 remove tough stems
6 eggs
2 spring onions, sliced (optional)
Handful of fresh coriander
 (optional)

1. Add the olive oil to a shallow pan with a lid and place over a medium heat.

2. Sweat the shallots in the pan with the green pepper, until the shallots are translucent and the pepper is tender.

3. Add the courgette and peas and continue to sweat. Then add 3 tablespoons of water and cover with the lid, until the vegetables are all soft.

4. Add the cumin, oregano, chilli flakes and salt and pepper, followed by the spinach and cavolo nero. Replace the lid, until the leaves have wilted and are tender.

5. Using the back of a spoon, create wells in the green mixture for the eggs to cook in. Carefully crack the eggs into the wells and replace the lid for 4–5 minutes, until the whites of the eggs have set and the yolks are still runny.

6. Top with the spring onions and coriander leaves, if using, and serve.

Apple and Banana Buckwheat Pancakes

Protein-packed and full of antioxidants to support your mitochondria, paired with a touch of natural sweetness, these outshine shop-bought pancakes and will be much more helpful for balancing blood-sugar levels, too. You'll never want to go back to traditional pancakes again.

Serves: 4
Total time: 20 minutes

100g buckwheat flakes
4 eggs (if you are vegan, use 1
  scoop of plant-based vanilla
  protein powder instead)
1 tsp cinnamon powder
1 banana, sliced in half
1 apple, cored and quartered
Coconut oil, for frying

Topping options (per pancake):
1 tbsp coconut yoghurt
1 tbsp desiccated coconut
Handful of fresh blueberries
Handful of fresh raspberries
1 tsp maple syrup

1. Blend the buckwheat flakes, eggs (or protein powder), cinnamon, banana and apple in a food processor. (If using protein powder, add 100ml water to combine.)

2. Heat 1 tsp coconut oil over a medium heat in a non-stick frying pan. Let the oil spread out evenly in the pan.

3. Once hot, pour in a ladle of the pancake mixture and move the pan around in a circular motion, until you have your desired shape and thickness.

4. Cook for 2–3 minutes before carefully flipping over and finishing off the other side for another minute or so. Reduce the heat if it gets too hot. Remove from the heat once the pancake is golden and brown. Transfer to a plate and keep warm while you cook the remaining pancakes.

5. Repeat steps 2–4 for the remaining batter and serve up with your chosen toppings.

Lunch

Miso-Baked Aubergine with Tenderstem Broccoli

Full of delicious umami flavours to really get your tastebuds working, this dish is the perfect lunch option. Miso paste packs a probiotic punch, while the aubergine and broccoli are rich sources of fibre, and the cashew nuts a great source of good fats and protein. Plus, antioxidants can be found in the skins of the aubergines (providing that rich purple hue). What's not to love?

Tip: pair this with a boiled egg for an added protein boost.

Serves: 2
Total time: 35 minutes

2 large aubergines, halved lengthways
Olive oil, for drizzling
1 heaped tbsp white miso paste
Juice of 1 lime

220g Tenderstem broccoli
70g cashew nuts
2 spring onions, diagonally sliced
Chilli flakes (optional)

1. Preheat the oven to 200°C.

2. Score a deep criss-cross on the flesh of the aubergines, without cutting through the skin. Drizzle some olive oil over both sides of the aubergine halves, then place skin-side up on a baking tray. Place in the oven for 10 minutes, then flip over the aubergines and return to the oven for a further 10 minutes.

3. Remove the aubergines from the oven and spread the miso paste evenly over each flesh half and squeeze over the lime juice, then return to the oven for a further 15 minutes, until the aubergines are soft throughout, and the miso is starting to turn thick and golden (keep an eye on them, as the miso is prone to burning quickly).

4. Meanwhile, blanch the broccoli in a pan of salted water for 3 minutes, then drain and set aside.

5. Toast the cashew nuts in a pan for 3–4 minutes over a medium–high heat, taking care not to burn them.

6. Serve the aubergines with the broccoli, spring onions and cashews, with a sprinkle of chilli flakes, if using.

Fluffy Egg and Chive Muffins

A great way to get protein and vegetables together in one neat little package, these savoury egg muffins will be an instant hit. Plus, they're a convenient way to get ahead when it comes to meal prep. Enjoy warm or cold.

Serves: 6
Total time: 30 minutes

Coconut oil (for greasing and frying)
1 whole broccoli head, chopped into small florets and stalks removed
Small pinch of chilli flakes (optional)
12 eggs
3 tbsp chives, finely chopped
7 sun-dried tomatoes, finely chopped
Salt and pepper

1. Preheat the oven to 200°C. Grease a 6-cup muffin tray with some coconut oil.

2. Heat 1 tbsp coconut oil in a frying pan and add the broccoli. Gently fry over a medium heat for 3–4 minutes, until al dente. Season with some salt, pepper and chilli flakes (if using).

3. Whisk the eggs in a bowl and add the chives and a sprinkle of salt and pepper.

4. Pour a thin layer of egg mixture into the base of each hole in the muffin tray. Then add some broccoli and sun-dried tomatoes to each. Repeat, until each hole is full and all the ingredients are used up.

5. Pop in the oven and bake for 20 minutes, until the muffins have risen and are cooked through, and golden and fluffy on the outside.

Asian Beef Mince Lettuce Boats

Bursting with Asian flavours, these beef mince lettuce boats are a real winner whenever you're lacking lunch inspiration. A perfect blend of protein, healthy fats and fresh vegetables, they are super quick and easy to make.

Serves: 4
Total time: 20 minutes
AIP-friendly

1 tsp coconut oil
400g beef mince
1 red onion, diced
2 tbsp grated ginger
6 baby button mushrooms, diced

1 carrot, grated
4 tbsp coconut aminos
1 avocado, diced into cubes
1–2 romaine lettuce hearts (or Chinese leaf)

1. Heat the coconut oil in a large frying pan over a high heat.

2. Add the beef mince and fry for about 8–10 minutes, stirring, until the beef is crispy and golden brown.

3. Reduce the heat slightly and add the red onion, grated ginger, mushrooms, carrot and coconut aminos and continue to cook through for a further 5 minutes, until everything has softened.

4. Divide the lettuce leaves between four plates and spoon over the mince mixture with the diced avocado on top.

Mackerel, Radish and Sweet Potato Poké Bowl

A delicious and nutritionally balanced lunch with a perfect trio of macronutrients (as well as being a rich source of omega-3 fats), teamed with a flavourful miso dressing. Yum!

Serves: 2
Total time: 20 minutes
AIP-friendly without the miso paste

1 sweet potato, cubed
1 tsp coconut oil
1 pak choi
1 carrot, peeled and grated
Handful of radishes, grated
2 fillets plain smoked mackerel (skinned and chopped into chunks)

1 spring onion, sliced
Handful of coriander, chopped

For the dressing:
1 tbsp coconut aminos
2 tsp white miso paste
Juice of ½ lime

1. Place the sweet potato cubes in a saucepan and pour over approximately 5cm of water, bringing to a boil and then simmering for 15 minutes. You may need to add a little more water as you go, depending on how dry the pan gets. Test with a fork to see if the potato is fully cooked, and then drain any remaining water from the pan.

2. Add the coconut oil to a frying pan and fry the pak choi leaves for 3–4 minutes, until softened and slightly golden.

3. Whisk the dressing ingredients together in a bowl.

4. Divide the carrot, radish, sweet potato, pak choi and mackerel between two poké bowls, followed by the spring onion and coriander, drizzling your dressing over the top.

Courgette and Sweetcorn Fritters

Courgette and sweetcorn offer a source of immuno-supportive vitamin C, while the eggs and chickpeas pack in protein and B vitamins. A healthy take on fritters, and great for maintaining energy levels throughout the day.

Serves: 2
Total time: 15 minutes

2 eggs

3 tbsp chickpea flour

1 courgette, grated

135g tinned sweetcorn, drained

2 tbsp fresh chives, finely
  chopped

½ tsp chilli flakes

1 tbsp coconut oil

Salt and pepper

Optional garnish:

2 handfuls of watercress

2 lemon wedges

1. Whisk the eggs together in a bowl. Gradually whisk in the chickpea flour, until you have a smooth batter.

2. Add the grated courgette, sweetcorn, chives, chilli flakes and salt and pepper and stir through.

3. Heat the coconut oil in a large, non-stick frying pan over a medium–high heat. Once the pan is hot, spoon out 2 tablespoons of batter into the pan to form a fritter. Repeat until you have filled the pan (you should be able to cook three or four at a time). Fry the fritters for 2–3 minutes, until they start to turn golden brown, then flip and repeat for a further 2 minutes, until cooked through.

4. Divide the fritters between two plates with a side of watercress and some lemon juice squeezed over, if desired.

Carrot and Coriander Soup

You can never go wrong with a nourishing homemade soup. Carrots are an excellent source of carotenoids (powerful antioxidants that provide the orange, yellow or red colour in certain plants). Coriander is also great for supporting heavy metal elimination. Pair this warming soup with a sprinkling of some nuts and seeds for an added protein and healthy-fat boost.

Serves: 3
Total time: 30 minutes
AIP-friendly

1 tsp coconut oil
1 onion, diced
570ml vegetable stock (source one that is AIP-friendly)

650g carrots, peeled and chopped
Handful of coriander

1. Melt the coconut oil in a large pan over a medium heat. Add the onion and fry for 5 minutes.

2. Pour in the vegetable stock, along with the carrots, and allow to simmer for 20 minutes, covered with a lid.

3. Once the carrots are soft, transfer the contents of the pan to a blender and blitz until smooth, adding more water if you prefer a less thick consistency.

4. Add the coriander to the blender and pulse for a further 5 seconds, just so it breaks up enough to mix through the soup. Serve immediately.

Vietnamese Prawn Summer Rolls

These are ideal for batch cooking and will keep in the fridge for two to three days. Jam-packed with nutrient-dense ingredients, including anti-inflammatory ginger, liver-supportive garlic and protein-packed prawns, these Vietnamese summer rolls will refresh the tastebuds and give you a midday pick-me-up.

Serves: 4
Total time: 40 minutes

100g brown rice noodles
½ red chilli, deseeded and
  finely chopped
2 garlic cloves, finely chopped
1 tbsp grated ginger
3 tbsp coconut aminos
Juice of 1 lime
8 brown rice paper sheets
  (22cm diameter)
7 jumbo cooked prawns (sliced
lengthways and then into
  small chunks)
1 carrot, peeled and cut into
  matchsticks
½ cucumber, cut into matchsticks
2–3 iceberg lettuce leaves,
  chopped
Handful of coriander leaves,
  finely chopped

1. Boil the rice noodles in a pan of hot water for 6–7 minutes or until cooked through.

2. Meanwhile, in a bowl, whisk together the chilli, garlic, ginger, coconut aminos and lime juice.

3. Drain the cooked noodles and add to the ginger and chilli dressing, stirring through. Cut through the noodles with a knife to allow for easier assembly of the rolls.

4. Pour some boiled water into a separate bowl. Taking one rice paper sheet at a time, immerse in the hot water for 15–20 seconds to soften, then gently place on a chopping board or other flat surface, taking care not to let the sides stick together.

5. Place 1 tablespoon of the noodles towards the bottom edge of a sheet, followed by a couple of pieces of prawn, some carrot sticks, cucumber, lettuce and coriander. Fold the left- and right-hand sides of the sheet towards the middle, followed by a small fold from the bottom edge. Now carefully and tightly roll with your filling three times to create your summer roll. Repeat with the remaining sheets and filling.

Beetroot and Chickpea Tabbouleh

Beetroot and quinoa are excellent sources of betaine (an amino acid that can support liver detoxification and the methylation cycle), while chickpeas can also help the methylation process as they are rich in folate (vitamin B9), as well as plant proteins.

Serves: 4
Total time: 20 minutes

150g quinoa
1 x 400g tin chickpeas, drained
200g radishes, grated
2 beetroots, grated
1 apple, cored and grated
25g flat-leaf parsley, chopped
25g mint, chopped
Juice of 2 lemons
2 tbsp olive oil
Generous pinch of salt and pepper

1. Add the quinoa to a saucepan with some hot water. Bring to the boil, then simmer for 10–15 minutes, until cooked through and soft. Drain and allow to cool in a sieve.

2. Meanwhile, combine the chickpeas, radishes, beetroots, apple, parsley and mint in a large mixing bowl and stir. Mix in the lemon juice and olive oil, along with the salt and pepper, and stir again.

3. Once the quinoa has cooled, stir into the tabbouleh and serve.

Greek Salad with Soft-Boiled Eggs

The Mediterranean diet is renowned for its health benefits and this classic Greek staple is no exception. It's refreshing, nutrient-dense and high in healthy monounsaturated fats. To make it dairy-free, I've replaced the feta with eggs to give you the perfect dose of protein. As well as being high in protein, egg yolks contain a compound called choline, which helps to regulate the nervous system.

Serves: 4
Total time: 10 minutes

4 eggs
1 cucumber
6 large vine tomatoes, each
  chopped into 8 pieces
1 green pepper, roughly
  chopped

1 small red onion, finely sliced
160g kalamata olives, pitted
2 tbsp olive oil
1 tbsp dried oregano
Generous pinch of salt

1. Place the eggs into boiling water over a high heat for 6 minutes.

2. Meanwhile, slice the cucumber in half lengthways. Using a teaspoon, gently scrape out the seeds and discard them, then chop the flesh into bite-sized chunks and place in a large salad bowl.

3. Add the remaining ingredients (apart from the eggs) and mix well.

4. Divide the salad equally between four bowls, then peel the eggs, slice them in half and serve one in each bowl.

Broccoli and Pak Choi Soup

Broccoli and pak choi are nutritional powerhouses, not least being excellent sources of chorophyll (the pigment that provides the green colour in vegetables, acting as a powerful antioxidant).

Tip: chlorophyll is fat-soluble, so why not add some healthy fats, such as a dollop of coconut yoghurt or nuts and seeds, to enhance absorption of this wonder compound?

Serves: 2
Total time: 20 minutes
AIP-friendly

1 tsp coconut oil
1 garlic clove, finely chopped
1 whole broccoli (including
  the stalk), chopped

570ml vegetable stock (source
  one that is AIP-friendly)
1 pak choi, chopped

1. Heat the coconut oil in a large pan. Add the garlic and fry over a medium heat for 2–3 minutes, until golden.

2. Add the chopped broccoli to the frying pan, along with the vegetable stock. Simmer over a medium heat, covered, for 10 minutes.

3. Add the pak choi to the pan, along with 300ml boiling water. Simmer, covered, for a further 5 minutes.

4. Pour the vegetable mixture into a blender and blend until smooth.

Dinner

Salmon and Vegetable Traybake

. . . .

A traybake is always a winner, saving on time when cooking for a family. Salmon is an amazing source of protein and healthy fats, and it's used here with polyphenol-rich vegetables that are full of fibre, vitamins and minerals, along with prebiotic fennel, onion and garlic (rather than using a shop-bought sauce). This dish takes things back to basics by simply using delicious herbs (giving you an extra dose of antioxidants), along with olives for that Mediterranean flavour. A firm favourite, no matter the season.

Serves: 2
Total time: 40 minutes
AIP-friendly

1 fennel bulb, roughly chopped
1 red onion, roughly chopped
1 courgette, sliced into rounds
160g kalamata olives, pitted
3–4 tbsp olive oil
1 tbsp oregano

2 salmon fillets
1 garlic clove, finely diced
1 broccoli head, chopped into
  mini florets
Handful of fresh basil leaves
Salt and pepper

1. Preheat the oven to 180°C.

2. Place the fennel, onion, courgette and olives on a large baking tray lined with baking parchment (you might need two if the vegetables do not fit).

3. Drizzle 2–3 tbsp olive oil over the vegetables and season with salt, pepper and the oregano. Give everything a mix and place in the oven for 30 minutes.

4. Meanwhile, lay the salmon fillets on another lined baking tray. Drizzle with a tablespoon of olive oil and sprinkle the garlic over the top of each fillet. Season with salt and pepper.

5. Fifteen minutes into the vegetable cooking time, place the salmon fillets in the oven and add the broccoli to the vegetables, mixing it through. Cook the salmon and vegetables for the remaining 15 minutes, until the salmon is cooked through and the vegetables are starting to soften and turn golden. Remove from the oven.

6. Sprinkle the basil leaves over the vegetables, divide between two plates and serve with the salmon.

Mediterranean Butterbean Stew

What's so great about this dish is that it's perfect for batch cooking – always recommended for CFS clients. You can prepare this dish on a Sunday evening and then it is ready to enjoy over the next few days. Simple and delicious.

Serves: 4
Total time: 50 minutes

1 red pepper
1 orange pepper
1 yellow pepper
1 tbsp coconut oil
1 onion, diced
3 garlic cloves, finely chopped
1 red chilli, deseeded and finely chopped
1 courgette, chopped into chunks
100g chargrilled artichokes, finely chopped
200g asparagus spears, halved
100g spinach
300ml vegetable stock
1 x 400g tin chopped tomatoes
½ tbsp oregano
1½ tbsp tomato purée
1 x 400g tin butter beans
Salt and pepper

1. Preheat the oven to 175°C.

2. Place the peppers on a lined baking tray and put in the oven for 30 minutes, until softened. The outer skin may also appear slightly black (this is ok, as you will peel it later).

3. Meanwhile, heat the coconut oil in a large frying pan over a medium heat. Add the onion and sauté for 2 minutes, until golden. You may need to add some water to the pan to prevent the onion from sticking.

4. Once the onion has softened, add the garlic, chilli, courgette, artichokes, asparagus and spinach and stir for 5 minutes over the medium heat.

5. Add the vegetable stock, tinned tomatoes, oregano and tomato purée. Bring to the boil and then simmer for 10 minutes.

6. Once the peppers have finished cooking, remove from the oven. Remove the skins and inner cores, then chop up the flesh with a knife (you might need to let them cool down for a couple of minutes before you do this).

7. Add the peppers and butter beans into the pan and continue to simmer for a further 15 minutes, lowering the heat if necessary.

8. Once the stew has finished cooking, season with salt and pepper and serve in individual bowls.

Ratatouille with Tender Chicken Thighs

Mouth-wateringly delicious, this ratatouille is paired here with succulent chicken thighs. Tomatoes are high in lycopene, an antioxidant that can protect our cells from oxidative damage.

Serves: 4
Total time: 35 minutes

1 tsp coconut oil
4 skinless and boneless
  chicken thighs
1 tsp olive oil
1 red onion, finely sliced
2 garlic cloves, finely chopped
1 large aubergine, sliced into

rounds (if the rounds get too
  big, slice them in half)
1 large courgette, sliced into
  rounds
2 beef tomatoes, chopped into
  wedges
1 x 400g tin plum tomatoes

250ml vegetable stock
1 tbsp oregano

2 tbsp fresh basil, finely
  chopped
Salt and pepper

1. Heat the coconut oil in a medium frying pan.

2. Once hot, add the chicken thighs and fry for 4–5 minutes, before turning and cooking the other side for the same time, until it has started to turn golden and brown (add a few tablespoons of water if the chicken begins to stick). Remove from the heat.

3. Meanwhile, heat the olive oil in a separate large frying pan. Add the onion and garlic and sweat for 3–4 minutes, until softened.

4. Add the aubergine and courgette and brown for 4 minutes, before adding the beef tomatoes, tinned plum tomatoes and vegetable stock. Add the oregano and basil, salt and pepper and simmer over a medium–high heat for 5 minutes, until the vegetables start to reduce.

5. Add the chicken thighs to the ratatouille and submerge. Cover with a lid and continue to simmer for another 10 minutes. Insert a skewer into the centre of the chicken – if the juices run clear, it is cooked through.

Vegeree

A vegetarian take on the famous kedgeree, this dish is abundant in micronutrients that will support energy levels, including B vitamin-rich brown rice and eggs, paired with anti-inflammatory spices to help fan the flames of chronic inflammation.

Serves: 4
Total time: 45 minutes

200g brown rice
1 tsp coconut oil
1 onion, diced

1 garlic clove, finely chopped
2 tsp ground coriander
½ tsp ground cumin

Seeds of 5 cardamom pods, crushed

1 tsp ground turmeric

1 tsp fresh grated ginger

1 small green chilli, deseeded and diced

4 eggs

1 yellow pepper, finely diced

1 courgette, diced

½ head of broccoli, chopped into tiny florets

50g kale

4 tbsp coconut yoghurt

60g sultanas

Juice of ½ lemon

Salt and pepper

Handful of parsley (optional)

Handful of flaked almonds (optional)

1. Fill a medium sized saucepan with boiling water and add the rice. Boil for 20–25 minutes.

2. Meanwhile, heat the coconut oil in a large pan over a medium heat. Fry the onion and garlic together for 3–4 minutes, until softened.

3. Add the ground coriander, cumin, cardamom seeds, turmeric, ginger and green chilli, stirring for 3 minutes.

4. Add the yellow pepper, courgette, broccoli and kale, and cook for 10 minutes, stirring through with the spices. Season with salt and pepper. If the pan starts to get dry, add a few tablespoons of water.

5. In a separate saucepan over a high heat, submerge the eggs into boiling water for 6 minutes for runny yolks (if you prefer firmer eggs, keep them in for a few minutes longer). Once boiled, shell the eggs and set aside.

6. Once the rice has cooked, drain well and mix into the pan with the vegetables and spices. Add the coconut yoghurt, sultanas and lemon juice, stirring everything through for a few more minutes.

7. Divide the rice between individual bowls with a boiled egg in each (sliced in half, so that the yolks ooze out). Season with salt and pepper and top with the parsley and flaked almonds, if using.

Kelp and Cabbage Stir-Fried Chicken Noodles

Iodine-rich kelp supports the production of thyroid hormones and is brought together with vitamin C-packed red cabbage and flavoursome chicken for a quick and easy stir-fry.

Serves: 2
Total time: 20 minutes
AIP-friendly

1 tsp coconut oil
2 chicken breast fillets, chopped into chunks
340g kelp noodles
1 thumb-sized stick of ginger, grated
1 carrot, peeled and grated

2 celery sticks, sliced
4 spring onions, sliced
¼ red cabbage, grated
2 tsp tamarind paste
4 tbsp coconut aminos
Handful of coriander

1. Heat the coconut oil in a medium-sized frying pan. Add the chicken-breast pieces and cook over a medium–high heat for 10–12 minutes, stirring, until it starts to brown.

2. Meanwhile, drain and rinse the kelp noodles.

3. Once the chicken has developed a crispy, golden appearance, add the ginger, carrot, celery, spring onions and cabbage, and fry for 3–4 minutes, until softened. You may want to add a splash of water to help the vegetables to soften slightly.

4. Add the kelp noodles, tamarind paste and coconut aminos, mixing everything through for a further 2 minutes.

5. Serve up with the coriander (**Note:** the noodles will still have a slight crunch when cooked).

Mexican-Spiced Turkey Tortillas with Sauerkraut

A protein-packed tortilla made entirely from chickpeas, served with turkey, fresh herbs and vegetables, and topped with probiotic-filled sauerkraut to provide a tangy punch and give your digestive system some love!

Serves: 2
Total time: 40 minutes

300g turkey mince
Coconut oil
3 tsp harissa paste (sugar-free)
150g chickpea flour
2 tbsp fresh chives, finely chopped
3 tbsp fresh parsley, finely chopped

100g coconut yoghurt
1 lime, quartered
100g cherry tomatoes, halved
1 baby romaine lettuce, chopped
2 spring onions, sliced
50g sauerkraut
Salt and pepper

1. Shape the turkey mince into 10 evenly sized balls and set aside on a plate.

2. Heat 1 tsp coconut oil in a frying pan over a medium–high heat. Add the meatballs, cooking for 10 minutes. Make sure that the outsides are golden and brown and that they are cooked right through. Add the harissa paste and stir together, before removing from the heat.

3. While the meatballs are frying, add the chickpea flour to a jug containing 170ml water. Add the chives and 2 tablespoons of parsley and stir through (adding a little more water if the chickpea mix starts to become too thick).

4. Mix the remaining parsley with the coconut yoghurt and squeeze in the juice from one lime wedge.

5. Heat 1 tsp coconut oil in a non-stick frying pan for each tortilla and bring to a high heat. Add a quarter of the chickpea mix and fry

for 1–2 minutes on each side, until golden and starting to crisp at the edges. Repeat three times to make a total of four tortillas.

6. Plate up the tortillas with a layer of yoghurt first, then add the meatballs, followed by the cherry tomatoes, romaine lettuce, spring onions and sauerkraut. Squeeze over the juice from the remaining lime wedges, season with salt and pepper and serve.

Coconut Fish Curry with Cauliflower Rice

Craving something warming and hearty for dinner? This coconut fish curry is jam-packed with nourishing ingredients and spices that will perk you up and provide heaps of flavour for your tastebuds, not to mention plenty of anti-inflammatory goodness.

Serves: 4
Total time: 50 minutes

2 tsp coconut oil
1 onion, diced
1 garlic clove, diced
1 red or green chilli, deseeded
  and diced
Seeds of 5 cardamom pods,
  crushed
1 tsp fennel seeds
2 tsp ground cumin
½ tsp ground turmeric, plus
  1 tsp for the cauliflower rice
Thumb-sized piece of fresh
  ginger, grated
½ tsp black peppercorn, crushed

1 x 400ml tin coconut milk
1 aubergine, cubed
200g cherry tomatoes, halved
Large handful of spinach
500g haddock loin, chopped
  into thumb-sized pieces
1 cauliflower, chopped into
  pieces
Salt and pepper
Handful of almonds, roughly
  chopped
Handful of fresh coriander,
  chopped

1. Heat 1 teaspoon of coconut oil in a pan over a medium–high heat. Add the onion, garlic and chilli and fry for 5 minutes.

2. Add the cardamom and fennel seeds, cumin, the half teaspoon of turmeric, ginger and crushed peppercorn and cook for another 5 minutes, adding a splash of water if the mixture starts to stick.

3. Add the coconut milk, along with the cubed aubergine, cherry tomatoes and spinach. Season with a generous pinch of sea salt, cover with a lid and simmer over a medium–high heat for 10 minutes.

4. Add the haddock pieces and simmer for a further 20 minutes, replacing the lid again.

5. Meanwhile, prepare the cauliflower rice by briefly pulsing the cauliflower into a rice-like consistency in a blender or food processor. You may want to do this in batches, as some food processors can only deal with small quantities at a time. Once you have achieved the desired consistency, heat the remaining coconut oil in a large pan and add the cauliflower rice. Sprinkle the teaspoon of ground turmeric in to create a yellow–orange hue and stir through, seasoning with some salt and pepper. Cook over a medium heat, for 10–15 minutes, stirring throughout, until the cauliflower rice is crispy and golden on the edges.

6. Serve the cauliflower rice with the fish curry in individual bowls, garnished with the chopped almonds and coriander.

Sesame Tempeh Summer Noodles with Ribboned Carrots and Mint

This nourishing mouth-watering dish is an absolute must for the summer months. Making ribboned carrots is the perfect way to get more vegetables into your diet without really noticing them! This dish captures so many Asian flavours – from the juicy lime and coconut aminos to the spice of chilli and ginger. It won't disappoint.

Serves: 2
Total time: 25 minutes

100g buckwheat noodles or
brown rice noodles
2 tsp sesame oil
1 red onion, finely sliced
250g carrots, sliced into
ribbons with a vegetable
peeler
160g tempeh, chopped into
cubes
1 red chilli, deseeded and diced

Thumb-sized piece of ginger,
grated
Handful of fresh mint leaves,
chopped

For the sauce:
3 tbsp coconut aminos
2 tbsp sesame seed oil
Juice of 1 lime
2 tbsp sesame seeds

1. Pour some boiling water into a pan over a high heat and cook the noodles for 10 minutes. Once softened, drain in a sieve.

2. Heat half the sesame oil in a frying pan, add the onion and fry for 4 minutes over a medium heat. Add the carrot ribbons, stirring for 5 more minutes, until soft.

3. Meanwhile, mix the sauce ingredients together in a small bowl.

4. In a separate frying pan, heat the remaining sesame oil over a medium–high heat, adding the tempeh and cooking for 2 minutes. Now add the chilli, ginger and half of the sauce, stirring for 2–3 minutes.

5. Add the drained noodles to the pan containing the carrots and onion and stir together. Pour over the remaining sauce and the chopped mint leaves.

6. Divide the noodle mixture between two bowls and serve with the tempeh mix on top.

Beef and Root Vegetable Stew with Rosemary and Thyme

Parsnips, leeks and carrots are full of fat-soluble nutrients (such as vitamin K) and are complemented with fresh rosemary, thyme and beef to add flavour and balance blood-sugar levels. Onion and garlic also support detoxification processes in the liver, making this a bowl of comforting nourishment. What more could you want?

Serves: 4
Total time: 1 hour 15 minutes
AIP-friendly

1 tsp coconut oil

1 large onion, diced

2 garlic cloves, finely chopped

1 litre beef stock or bone broth (source one that is AIP-friendly)

1 tbsp fresh thyme leaves, chopped

2 tbsp fresh rosemary sprigs

800g stewing beef, diced

3 carrots, peeled and halved lengthways, then cut into chunks

2 parsnips, peeled and halved lengthways, then cut into chunks

3 leeks, sliced into rounds

1. Heat the coconut oil in a stewing pot or large saucepan over a medium heat. Add the onion and garlic and sweat for a couple of minutes.

2. After no more than 5 minutes, pour in the beef stock and stir in the thyme and rosemary. Bring to the boil, then add the diced beef, carrots, parsnips and leeks. Cover with a lid and simmer over a medium–low heat for 1 hour, stirring once halfway through.

3. Serve the stew in individual bowls.

Chicken, Basil and Courgette Skewers

Moist chicken thighs marinated in a lemon and basil dressing and served on a skewer with delicious veggies. Super versatile, accompanied with any side of your choosing.

Serves: 2
Total time: 45 minutes
AIP-friendly

½ butternut squash, peeled and deseeded, then cut into skewer-sized cubes
2 tbsp olive oil
2 tbsp dried basil
Juice of 1 lemon
Generous pinch of salt
2 large chicken thighs (skinless and boneless), cut into cubes

2 red onions, sliced into 4cm pieces
2 courgettes, sliced into rounds
2 handfuls of rocket (optional)

You will also need:
8–10 25cm wooden or metal skewers (if using wooden skewers, soak in water before cooking)

1. Preheat the oven to 180°C.

2. Boil the butternut squash cubes in 5cm of water for 7 minutes, until al dente. You don't want them to become too soft – just enough that you can easily get a skewer through them.

3. Whisk together the olive oil, dried basil, lemon juice and salt in a large mixing bowl, until combined. Add the chicken, red onions, courgette and squash and mix through, leaving to marinate for 5–10 minutes.

4. Thread the chicken pieces, courgettes, onion and squash on to skewers until they are all full. Place on a baking tray and cook in the oven for 10 minutes, then turn the skewers and cook the other side for a further 10 minutes, until the chicken and vegetables are starting to brown slightly and the chicken is white in the middle. Remove and serve with some rocket, if using.

Suggested Meal Plan

	Monday	**Tuesday**	**Wednesday**
Breakfast	Buckwheat Bircher Muesli with Grated Carrot and Pear	Fluffy Egg and Chive Muffin leftovers, with sautéed spinach, olive oil and salt	Coconut and Flax Turmeric 'Porridge' with Stewed Apple
Lunch	Fluffy Egg and Chive Muffin, served with rocket and sauerkraut	Miso-Baked Aubergine with Tenderstem Broccoli and leftover traybake vegetables	Carrot and Coriander Soup, sprinkled with broccoli sprouts and crushed walnuts, served with two oatcakes and houmous
Dinner	Salmon and Vegetable Traybake	Kelp and Cabbage Stir-Fried Chicken Noodles	Mexican-Spiced Turkey Tortillas with Sauerkraut

Thursday	Friday	Saturday	Sunday
Kiwi and Spinach Chia Pudding	Leftover Kiwi and Spinach Chia Pudding, sprinkled with coconut flakes	Leafy-Green Shakshuka, served with kimchi	Apple and Banana Buckwheat Pancakes with coconut yoghurt and fresh berries
Vietnamese Prawn Summer Rolls	Greek Salad with Soft-Boiled Eggs and two oatcakes, topped with half a sliced avocado and chilli flakes	Asian Beef Mince Lettuce Boats	Courgette and Sweetcorn Fritters
Vegeree	Sesame Tempeh Summer Noodles with Ribboned Carrots and Mint	Coconut Fish Curry with Cauliflower Rice	Ratatouille with Tender Chicken Thighs

CHAPTER 15

Lifestyle I – Energy Management

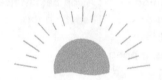

Patience is bitter, but its fruit is sweet.
Jean-Jacques Rousseau, Genevan philosopher,
writer and composer

In this section, we will cover the various lifestyle tools that you can incorporate into your daily routine to support recovery from CFS.

Let's begin with an in-depth look at energy, rest and activity management.

The importance of energy management

We all require energy to undertake tasks both physical and mental in nature. Energy also fuels our internal functions, such as body temperature and metabolism (known as our basal metabolic rate, or BMR for short). Our cells need energy to repair, build and maintain bodily tissues; for instance, if we become injured, our cells require energy to flood white blood cells towards the wound.

The common denominator in CFS is a limited supply of energy to meet the body's basic needs, worsened by any form of physical, mental or emotional exertion. The decline in energy supply means that even basic tasks can result in prolonged fatigue and brain fog. Daily life becomes a constant reminder of what you used to be able to do, underlining the harsh reality of your current capacity. This stark shift presents its own challenges, but it also highlights potential for progress: your energy balance may have taken a bit of a hit, but it doesn't need to stay this way for ever.

The process of energy management is one of trial and error. You implement something to see if it goes well or not. If it doesn't, you know to taper things back next time; and if it does, that's great, and you can continue with the strategy.

A sense of awareness is particularly useful before you start to look at how you can change your daily activities to help with your fatigue. I have had many clients come to me and say that they cannot identify what in their routines has led to an increase in fatigue. Often, this is because they are comparing themselves to when they were fully functioning. Some people say that they have 'done nothing all day', even though they have showered, tidied the house, washed the dishes, taken their dog for a short walk and prepared meals. It is easy to discount these everyday jobs, and even the mental or emotional tasks that can drain your energy reserves, too. I would encourage you to become more aware of your daily habits and the energy that is required to do all the things you do.

Navigating energy management

When it comes to navigating your recovery from CFS, you will need to give careful consideration towards three distinct factors:

- The stage of illness you are in (the 'crash', 'wired-and-tired' or 'restoration' stage)
- Severity of your symptoms (mild, moderate or severe)
- The extent to which your illness fluctuates daily (this might be due to PEM or an exacerbation)

What is the difference between PEM and an exacerbation?
PEM is an abnormal response to exertion (also known as activity intolerance). It involves a worsening of symptoms and a reduction in stamina and functional capacity, which can be triggered by physical, emotional

or mental activity. It may also be prompted by standing up after periods of sitting, which is common in those who suffer with PoTS (postural orthostatic tachycardia syndrome – an abnormal increase in heart rate after sitting up or standing).

PEM can be delayed by a day or two after the trigger activity and, in some cases, recovery time can last from days to weeks. The longer or more physically demanding the activity, the worse PEM is likely to be. Plus, if you continue to overexert yourself soon after experiencing PEM, this may also contribute to a worsening of symptoms.

An exacerbation is a worsening in CFS symptoms, not because of exercise or activity but due to:

- catching an infection
- eating a food that you are sensitive or intolerant to
- environmental triggers such as sounds, lights, toxic chemicals, vaccinations and extreme temperature changes
- physical trauma (say, a car accident, surgery, childbirth)

Exacerbations and PEM can occur at any stage on the road to recovery and I often advise keeping a diary of common triggers for these. That way, you can identify a pattern of what is regularly causing your symptoms to crash (**Note:** a symptom crash is not necessarily the same as the crash stage of CFS).

What is meant by 'rest'?

When you think about the word 'rest', what comes to mind? Maybe it's sitting on the sofa watching your favourite TV programme? Or having an afternoon snooze? For our purposes, the word 'rest' can be defined as either:

- stopping work or movement to relax or recover strength
- allowing yourself to be inactive to regain health and energy.

These definitions imply that the purpose of resting is to achieve relaxation and, ultimately, to recover your health and energy. Therefore, focus on the *quality* of rest that you take, so that you don't hinder your recovery. While one part of resting is being physically still or 'inactive', what ultimately determines good-quality rest is the relaxation part (we will cover ways to support this on pp. 254–256).

Different types of rest include:

- bed rest
- rests during the day
- mental rest
- sleep.

Physical forms of rest involve sitting down, standing still or lying down. But mental rest is also very important here because this is what determines the quality of any form of physical rest, so that it becomes relaxing and, ultimately, restorative.

Rest is particularly important during the early stages of CFS (i.e. the 'crash' stage), as well as at times when you experience PEM or any exacerbations of the illness. Rest is also important to help prevent an increase in symptoms, so it's not just a means of recovery from a crash.

Exercise vs physical activity

Exercise is any form of movement that is focused upon improving physical fitness (running or lifting weights, for example), whereas physical activity is any bodily movement in which there is use of the muscles (such as making the bed, standing up or emptying the dishwasher). While there is some overlap between the two, and exercise *is* a form of physical activity, not all physical activity can be classed as exercise (for example, emptying the dishwasher).

In the earlier days of recovery, you should just aim for physical activity, as you start to build up your tolerance towards exercise once again. (We will look at activity management and exercise in more detail on pp. 235–239.)

Steering through the 'crash' stage

At the crash stage, fatigue will be at an all-time high and your mood will be at an all-time low.

This is the earliest stage of CFS, when you may well be on bed rest, which is encouraged initially during the acute phase of illness (or during any severe exacerbations). However, there can be some negative effects on the body if it is inactive for too long (these are covered below and on the next page). That's why it's important to recognise when your body is able to tolerate a mild activity level, such as getting out of bed and sitting in a chair or walking slowly – but this should only happen when some form of recovery progress has started to take place.

I know how frustrating the crash stage can be. During this time, aim for good-quality sleep, stay calm and accept your body's current situation by telling yourself that 'this too shall pass'. Yes, it can feel like an endless waiting game for the fatigue to alleviate, but don't fight the process.

An adequate period of rest during this early stage can be a way to reduce the severity of the illness, which could be worsened if you push and force yourself to exercise too early on in the illness.

The drawbacks of prolonged rest

Being inactive for too long can cause changes in the capacity of the lungs and heart, as well as blood-pressure changes and muscle wastage (loss of muscle mass and strength). Even small amounts of movement can be supportive if long periods of inactivity are still a necessary part of your resting routine.

To ensure that you don't experience muscle wasting due to deconditioning from long periods of being immobile, try to perform some gentle limb movements.

Start by flexing and relaxing your feet and toes. You might then want to build up towards squeezing and releasing your fists and glute muscles, and even some gentle hip abduction (moving the legs away from the midline of the body), if you can. Although small movements, these can be significant in getting your muscles moving again.

When you start to feel a little stronger, see if you can get your body to sit upright, slowly increasing the time that you do this for. Next, see if you can sit in a chair and then, eventually, stand or gently move about the house for a short while. Be on the lookout for signs of overdoing it – your body should give you some feedback, and you might start to feel more tired. If so, just ease up on the activity and continue to rest, until you feel up to some gentle and restorative movement again.

The crash stage: In a nutshell
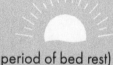

Physical and mental rest (including an initial period of bed rest) are essential during the crash stage, until you start to see signs of symptom improvement. At this point, mild physical activity should be slowly and carefully attempted again.

Steering through the 'wired-and-tired' stage

In this stage of recovery, you are starting to see some signs that your energy is rebuilding. However, this type of energy is not serving you well because a lot of it is going towards the nervous system (see p. 45). So although some energy is returning to the body, rather than feeling vigour you are still prone to feeling exhausted. Many of my clients describe themselves in this stage as feeling wired (hence the name of this stage), jittery and anxious, with levels of brain fog very high. There is almost a sense of running on adrenaline, yet at the same time energy levels are on the floor – it's a real mixed bag of feelings.

There will likely be an initial increase in physical capacity compared with the crash stage, which is why it is recommended to start to explore physical activity at a pace that the body can handle (see guidance on pacing on p. 221 and grading on p. 225).

PEM is likely to be more evident in this stage of recovery because this is the first time you will be having a real go at undertaking physical activity (and possibly exercise) once again (whereas the crash stage involved much more rest). This is the classic scenario of 'boom and bust' (see p. 222).

The wired-and-tired stage: In a nutshell

There is an increase in physical capacity during this stage, but fatigue is still very much present, with most people feeling 'wired and tired'. I recommend gradually introducing physical activity (and exercise only if and when the body can handle it) because levels of PEM may be high.

Pacing is very important during this stage to help settle the nervous system down and get your energy to rebalance within the body, helping you to reach the 'restoration' stage of recovery.

Steering towards the 'restoration' stage

At this stage, you are not feeling wired and tired so much and your nervous system has started to calm down. You should now have some solid evidence that your baseline level of activity has increased, you are capable of more physical and mental activities and PEM and exacerbations are getting less and less frequent. You may find that you are slowly starting to do some of the things that you used to do previously, but there is an awareness that you are still not at the same level of functional capacity as you were pre-CFS.

Recovery at this stage is all about continuing pacing and grading (see below and p. 225) and focusing on how far you have come, while working on emotional-energy drainers or niggling physical ones. Consider how much emotional energy you are spending on things. This could be worrying about your health, relationship difficulties, work or financial stresses or simply biting off more than you can chew. Can you see how these mental factors might tax your energy on a physical level and hold you back from optimum health?

The restoration stage: In a nutshell

PEM and exacerbations are becoming less and less frequent. Continue pacing and grading and focus on reducing any physical and emotional energy drainers that are still holding you back – but always make sure you celebrate how far you have come.

What is pacing?

Pacing is one of the key principles that I teach CFS clients. It is also being used by the NHS for supporting CFS and, more recently, long-COVID patients. But what is pacing? And how do you know if you are doing it right?

Pacing is an energy-management strategy that seeks to find the balance between activity and rest. It involves living within the physical and mental limits imposed by illness and avoiding physical and mental activities that exacerbate symptoms. Pacing may also involve implementing scheduled rests around any form of activity undertaken. To pace, you must carefully evaluate your daily activities and get them to a level that your body can handle, based upon where you are on the road to recovery.

Pacing is very important at all stages of recovery (but particularly in the wired-and-tired stage, when it becomes possible to reintroduce activity). I always tell clients they will never get it right 100 per cent of the time, but it's a process of understanding past hiccups, when they might have 'overdone it', and tapering things back to a comfortable place – one that supports energy flowing back into the body again to build up reserves (see the next page for more on this).

The boom-and-bust cycle

Even with the limited energy capacity that characterises CFS, on better days, when you feel a little bit more energy coming in than usual, you may tend to get excited and eager to do as much as you possibly can. I've seen this time and time again with clients and have even been guilty of it myself.

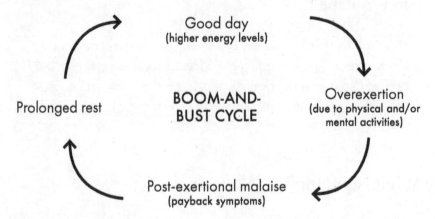

Good day
(higher energy levels)

Prolonged rest

BOOM-AND-BUST CYCLE

Overexertion
(due to physical and/or mental activities)

Post-exertional malaise
(payback symptoms)

The boom-and-bust cycle is a seemingly natural pattern for many with CFS, whereby they overdo it on the good days and only end up resting when there is no choice – when their batteries are completely flat, and they have no option but to let them recharge.

I always say, you know your body much better than me, as you are the one who's living in it. But the experience you have had from PEM is teaching you something – that you need to ease off on pushing your nervous system and let go of that sense of urgency around getting back to full capacity.

But how do you do this? Well, it is all about using smaller amounts of energy and breaking down tasks, with time to rest in between (for example doing three fifteen-minute sessions of cleaning – morning, afternoon and evening – rather than forty-five minutes in one go).

As an example, you might normally get up, shower, brush your teeth, get dressed and make your bed, all within a period of ten to fifteen minutes. If you are pacing, however, you might space out these tasks with a buffer to rest in between each one. You might sit down and rest for five minutes after your shower and consider making your bed at another time during the day, for example. By chunking basic tasks down with room to rest in between, you are rationing your energy more effectively, so that your body has some 'charging' time to build up its energy reserves and the likelihood of crashing is reduced.

Prioritise the important stuff

Try to prioritise more important tasks or, alternatively, enlist the support of a friend or family member who is understanding of your current situation and can help you with the essential things, like cooking or housework, for instance.

If there is an important event coming up that you know is going to tax your energy, give yourself some leeway and wiggle room to breathe. This might involve scheduling in some 'you' time to rest, both before *and* after the event, or in case you experience PEM afterwards. This will help to ensure that your battery supply is sufficient for other upcoming activities, plus it helps to build up reserves for an emergency.

Follow the 75-per-cent rule

When dealing with CFS, it's important to budget your energy in a similar way to your finances, taking care not to use more than you can afford.

I encourage clients to follow the 75-per-cent rule, which involves staying within 75 per cent of your energy envelope and not stretching above and beyond this. This tends to involve some intuition, trial and error and listening to your body. You need to find your baseline (the point at which your symptoms start to increase following any changes in activity levels – more of which on the next page) and then drop your activity level back by 25 per cent, to the point where symptoms ease off and stay that way for a few days. Becoming more in tune with minor symptoms that are more pronounced upon increased exertion/activity can help with pre-empting this.

The 75-per-cent rule is therefore about easing up enough to allow some breathing room for your energy reserves to recoup.

Find your baseline

Your baseline is the level of activity (physical, mental or both) that you can comfortably manage on at least three to four consecutive days, without experiencing symptoms as a result. It often begins as less than you would imagine, but do not be discouraged by this.

Once you have established your baseline, keep to this amount of activity for at least two weeks as a safety measure to ensure that you do not experience any PEM. Settle into it and try to accept that this is where you and your body are at right now.

Let's use a client of mine, Rebecca, as an example. This was her baseline daily level of activity during the wired-and-tired stage:

- Shower
- Make the bed
- 1.5-mile dog walk
- Twenty minutes social media (ten minutes in the morning and ten in the evening)
- Ten minutes checking e-mails
- One hour watching Netflix (always something light-hearted, like a comedy)
- Fifteen-minute online yoga class
- Ten minutes journaling

Rebecca could achieve these activities for the distances or durations described above as her baseline each day. However, if she did any more than this, she experienced PEM.

If you look at the first graph on p. 225, you'll see that there were peaks and troughs in Rebecca's energy levels (aka boom and bust), based upon how far she veered from her baseline activity levels.

Now look at the second graph. By adopting the 75-per-cent rule, Rebecca was able to increase her baseline over time, meaning that an increased level of activity became possible for her without experiencing PEM. Energy is starting to increase at a stable and steady rate, which is where activity (and recovery) progress can be made.

Maintain, progress, maintain!

Introducing new levels of activity should be done slowly and by listening to the body and its capacities. Grading is an approach that involves gradually increasing your activity level, while allowing time to see if your body can maintain that level before implementing further changes. When you start to introduce grading, you only apply the 75-per-cent rule again if PEM or an exacerbation occur. By grading up, you are gradually 'raising the bar', the idea being to maintain a newly achieved baseline for two weeks, then to progress (in other words 'grade' activity), then maintain that for two weeks and so on.

In Rebecca's case, this meant increasing her dog walk from 1.5 to 2 miles and either staying with that for two weeks if no PEM arose (this would be her new baseline) or tapering back to 1.5 miles if it did. In the event that PEM arose as a result of grading, the next stage would involve trying a middle ground of 1.75 miles (once she was feeling up to it) and so on. The third and fourth graphs show a comfortable progression of Rebecca's baseline.

It is normal to experience the odd dip in symptoms (which sometimes have their own wicked way), but it won't be like before in the boom-and-bust pattern, and you will be more in control. Slow and steady really does win the race.

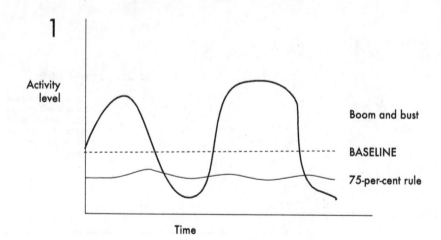

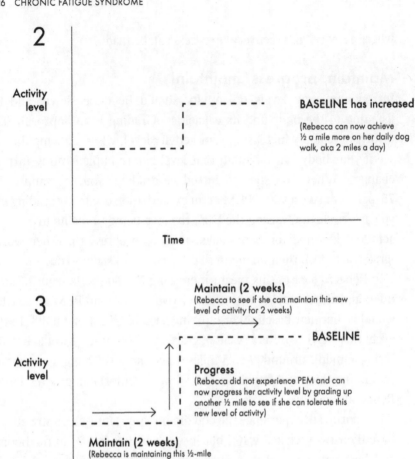

2

Activity level

BASELINE has increased

(Rebecca can now achieve ½ a mile more on her daily dog walk, aka 2 miles a day)

Time

3

Maintain (2 weeks)
(Rebecca to see if she can maintain this new level of activity for 2 weeks)

BASELINE

Activity level

Progress
(Rebecca did not experience PEM and can now progress her activity level by grading up another ½ mile to see if she can tolerate this new level of activity)

Maintain (2 weeks)
(Rebecca is maintaining this ½-mile activity level increase for 2 weeks to see if she experiences PEM)

Time

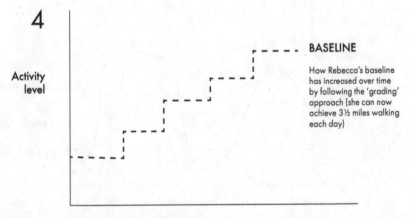

4

BASELINE

Activity level

How Rebecca's baseline has increased over time by following the 'grading' approach (she can now achieve 3½ miles walking each day)

Time

In essence, pacing is all about living within the imposed limits of the illness and finding your baseline, whereas grading (physical, mental or both) over time is about expanding your energy envelope as you move forwards in the recovery journey. There is quite a close relationship between the two, the goal being that you are both pacing and increasing your activity tolerance at the same time.

Set realistic goals

It can be helpful to focus on what you can do as part of your baseline, and then, over time, compare this with things that are not currently within your reach. Focusing mostly on what you *can* do can be so empowering as you will start to see, as recovery progresses, how you're achieving things you previously couldn't. Even if you feel like you have nothing to put into the left-hand column (below), activities that you consider to be minor are still worth noting:

What I can do right now	What I would like to be able to do
Brush teeth	Walk up and down the stairs
Lift head from pillow	Leave the house
Sit in a chair for ten minutes each day	Walk around the house
Eat three meals and put plates by the door	Shower myself
Use the bathroom	Socialise
Read for ten minutes	Do my job

Keep an activity diary

With awareness being a key focus of energy management, complete a diary, listing the various activities you have done throughout the day, while rating your symptoms in relation to each one. A task can be:

- energy-building – i.e. it gives you energy
- energy-neutral – i.e. it neither builds nor drains your energy
- energy-draining – i.e. it drains your energy and makes you feel tired.

Remember, these don't always have to be physical activities – they can be mental or emotional, too.

Here is an example of how you might set out an activity diary:

Activity (physical/ mental/emotional)	Symptoms rating (out of 10, where 0 is the best, 10 is the worst it could be)	Is the task energy-building/neutral/ draining?
Walk in the park	Physical fatigue 6/10	Energy-draining
On Instagram (ended up comparing myself to my friends having a good time)	Physical fatigue 7/10 – felt physically tired twenty minutes later	Energy-draining
Hoovering the house	Physical fatigue 8/10	Energy-draining
Drinking a cup of tea	N/A	Energy-neutral
Watching a nature documentary on TV	N/A	Energy-building
Meditating	N/A	Energy-building
Medical appointment	Physical fatigue 7/10 and brain fog soon afterwards 9/10	Energy-draining

Have a go yourself at completing the diary opposite at home.

Remember that this is all context dependent, and the same task could be energy-building on one day and energy-draining the next. Take watching TV, for example – a nature documentary could be relaxing and therefore energy-building, whereas a horror film could be energy-draining. In fact, the same documentary could have different effects on different days, depending on whether you are relaxed or stressed.

- When you have done this exercise for a week, think about whether your responses depended on . . .
  - when you were doing the activity (time of day)
  - whether your symptoms were flaring that day
  - where you were doing the activity

Activity (physical/ mental /emotional)	Symptoms rating (out of 10, where 0 is the best, 10 is the worst it could be)	Is the task energy-building/neutral/ draining?

- – whether you were standing or sitting
- – whether you were stressed or feeling emotional
- – whether other people were supporting you during the activity.

Completing a diary considering the above should help you to spot daily changes in your energy based on the activities that you do. If you find you have too many energy-draining tasks compared with either energy-building or energy-neutral ones, this is a sign that you need to change things to achieve a better energy balance. (Aim for at least three energy-building tasks each day and either shorten the duration of the energy-draining tasks or avoid them altogether, depending on how essential they are to daily living.)

Switching

Switching involves changing up activities to avoid tiring out specific muscles. By trying short periods of different types of activity in this way, certain parts of your body can rest, while others are working. For example, if you have been reading, stop before your eye muscles get tired and try something that involves a different muscle group. This might be talking, walking or some gentle stretching. Do this next activity for a little while and then switch to another one. Choose between a few physical and mental tasks, interspersed with rest breaks to reduce the impact of your activities on your energy. For example:

- Ten minutes of cleaning – physical activity
- Twenty minutes of meditation (seated in an armchair) – mental and physical rest
- Fifteen minutes reading emails on the computer – mental activity

A rest break can also mean switching activity, rather than complete rest, depending on how you feel – say, walking about the house, putting on some relaxing music, drinking some water, stretching or doing the opposite of what you have been doing in that moment.

Ⅱ

Improving brain fog

Did you know that your brain is responsible for around 20 per cent of your body's daily energy expenditure? That's a lot of energy needed to power our thinking caps!

Because brain function is so energy demanding, it makes sense that in CFS, certain cognitive tasks can be draining, resulting in feelings of both physical and mental fatigue. In fact, brain fog itself is a symptom of energy deficiency in the brain. This can occur even if you have some physical energy present in CFS, but you experience mental fatigue as your most prominent symptom.

So what can be done to support the symptoms of mental fatigue?

- **Don't multi-task**. Multi-tasking can scatter attention and impair cognitive function and memory, as you become more easily distracted and impulsive when completing multiple tasks at once. Try to stick to one task at a time (whether physical or mental), allowing your brain the chance to focus itself, rather than drain its batteries.

- **Write lists**. These can be handwritten to-do lists or notes on your computer. This will help you to remember things and keep all your ducks in a row, so to speak.

- **Keep a 'minutes of meeting' if you have returned to work**. If you are on a phased return to work, keep a written 'minutes of meeting', so that you can remember the salient points from discussions in meetings.

- **Be honest and open**. Express your concerns about your brain symptoms to family members and colleagues.

> • **Pace yourself**. Ensure that you take short breaks throughout the day to function better.

Give yourself permission to rest

Resting can help you to fill up your cup, so that the body can function optimally and undertake daily activities. But seldom do we give ourselves permission to have some down time.

Make rest a priority, even if you don't think you need it. In the same way that a doctor would write a prescription for medication, write yourself a prescription for rest.

It can be tempting to fight against resting, but this can often make things worse. Listen to your body and give yourself permission. Really allowing yourself to decompress and rest, both mentally and physically – without getting eaten up by guilt or feeling that you are 'giving in' to your illness – will improve the overall quality of rest, which, in turn, will help with energy production in the body. And remember:

*It is not that you are no longer **capable** – it is just that your **capacity** has changed, and this can improve over time.*

So don't beat yourself up about the odd nap here and there; instead, reframe it as a 'recharge' – a non-negotiable that will set you up for a more productive day ahead.

Also, know that it is ok to cancel plans if you do not have the energy or to say no to things that energetically you cannot afford; otherwise, your health will be negatively affected.

For more advice on how to switch off and find a sense of calm within mind and body, see pp. 254–257.

Healing your perspective on fatigue

When it comes to tiredness, it's important to understand that not all fatigue is the same or arises from the same factors.

It can be all too easy to get caught up in thinking that CFS is to blame for your tiredness, but remember that fatigue is a beast that rears its ugly head for everyone, and you are bound to experience it at various stages in your life, irrespective of your condition. As one client said to me, 'Sometimes my husband will say to me, "I'd be tired today, too, if I had done X." It can be a humble reminder that sometimes we do things that would make anyone feel run-down or burnt out.'

A few types of tiredness to put this into context:

- **Emotional tiredness** – mental and emotional reactions to life events can result in bodily fatigue and exhaustion, as mental capacity becomes strained.

- **Physical tiredness** – you've used up more energy than your body can create during this moment. You may also have an underlying medical concern that is driving symptoms of physical fatigue, which may not be CFS-related.

- **Environmental tiredness** – this is the name for tiredness arising from doing one thing for too long (i.e. without taking breaks), not breathing correctly, lack of food, water, fresh air or exercise. Our bodies are designed to move, breathe and take breaks and, when this doesn't happen, a feeling of tiredness is normal.

JOSHUA, AGED THIRTY-FIVE

Joshua is currently in the wired-and-tired stage of his recovery, which means that he has transitioned from the crash stage and some energy is coming back into his body; however, he is still prone to feeling exhausted and experiences the effects of the boom-and-bust cycle (see p. 222). This is why a lot of the work that Joshua and I have done together has involved sensible pacing, with a real focus on him becoming attuned towards listening to his body systems and what they are communicating to him.

I asked Joshua to complete an activity diary so that we could ascertain which patterns in his life were energy-building, energy-draining or energy-neutral, to ensure that he spends most of his time performing the energy-building or energy-neutral activities. He found this to be a gamechanger in understanding what leaves holes in his energy bucket, so that he could reduce PEM and crashes. Joshua also followed the 75-per-cent rule, which enabled him to build up his baseline over time, as he then progressed his levels of activity, while resting in between. As he says:

'I have learned the art of allowing my body to rest. I am aware of the activities that reduce my energy, as well as those which charge up my battery. I can now plan my life sensibly to reduce the likelihood of crashing. For example, if I have something coming up in my diary that runs the risk of me crashing, I look to make sure that my schedule is filled with energy-building activities (such as meditation, yoga and gardening), so that I can build up tolerance ahead of the event, and recharge when it's over.'

CHAPTER 16

Lifestyle II – Exercise, Physical Activity and Recovery

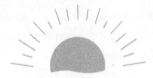

He who has health has hope, and he who has hope has everything.
Thomas Carlyle, Scottish essayist

Physical movement can support mood, concentration and sleep; therefore, it is important to incorporate some activity (even if it is very minimal to start with), without triggering PEM. Alongside pacing and other strategies we've looked at, physical activity can be used therapeutically if it is carefully managed and structured at the right stage of the recovery journey.

Gentle forms of physical activity are recommended in the early stages of CFS, only when the body feels able (see 'The crash stage', on the next page). However, when it comes to exercise, this must be approached with extreme caution in CFS. In fact, you may run the risk of worsening your illness if you overdo it too early on. Only when your body is showing positive signs of recovery should you begin to recondition your muscles. Remember, one of the hallmarks of CFS is PEM (also known as 'activity intolerance'), which is why you need to be very careful about how you navigate exercise and any form of activity when recovering.

- **The crash stage:** listen to your body intently during this stage and only incorporate light physical activity when the body allows. Think gentle limb movements, walking around the house, standing up and sitting down, yin yoga and some light stretching.

- **The wired-and-tired stage:** during this stage, your body is likely to be more tolerant of physical activity, and exercise may finally be on the horizon. Adopt the principles of grading (as discussed on p. 225), which involves increasing your activity, then maintaining it for a period before attempting another increase. It helps to think of grading as being like a staircase, rather than a slope. If and when your body allows, start to incorporate low-intensity exercise (while still following the principles of grading), such as swimming, cycling, Pilates, hatha yoga, brisk walking or some light jogging. Be wary of the boom-and-bust pattern (see p. 222), be mindful and, as always, listen to your body.

- **The restoration stage:** you may find that your nervous system has started to calm down and, as a result, you might feel able to introduce exercises that are higher in impact or intensity (for example, running, high-intensity interval training, boxing or weights). While these can indeed be a possibility for you again, do continue to follow the principles of grading, implementing movements mindfully and sensibly, while remembering those activities that are gentler and more restorative on the nervous system and that can support recovery. If you find that impactful forms of exercise are still not possible for you, continue to pace and be patient with your body and its current capacities.

Note: any activity-management regime that emphasises either too much rest or too forceful a return to physical activity and/or exercise (particularly in the early stages) is unsafe.

Increase the duration of exercise (before the intensity)

Once you have established your baseline for activity, you can try to increase the duration. This is often better and more appropriate than increasing the activity level, simply because the body can more easily pace itself to withstand longer levels of activity than push itself to a higher capacity. So when your body feels able, gently increase activity duration by 10 per cent, wait two weeks to assess for any PEM and, if there isn't any, experiment again with another 10 per cent and so on.

This helps to build your reserves so that you can expand on it as your health improves. Any sudden or intense activity will almost certainly lead to a crash, so try to follow a grading regime that listens to your body and where it is at. Do not allow anyone to push you any further than you feel comfortable with – including yourself or any health professionals.

If there is a crash, you might need to reduce or completely stop the exercise you are doing. If so, use this as a time to pause, reflect and identify any triggers that might have incited the crash, helping you to plan accordingly and make any appropriate adaptations to your routine moving forwards. It is all about balancing the energy equilibrium.

If you are experiencing a progressive degree of recovery, which involves very few crashes or PEM, this is a good indication that you can continue to gradually increase your periods of physical and mental activity, while reducing the time you spend resting.

Healing your relationship with exercise

Sometimes we associate our symptoms with exercise and become fearful of integrating it back into our routines. But seeing your body tolerate more activity is proof positive that you are on the right track. So try to deal with any fear around exercise and how to approach it safely, remembering that what hurt you in the past may not hurt you now. Things like journaling or EFT (see pp. 276 and 280) can be helpful here, or you might consider seeking professional support to get yourself into a better mindset for dealing with any blocks around introducing exercise.

LIZZIE, AGED TWENTY-NINE

When I first became unwell with CFS, I was sleeping for four hours during the day due to pure exhaustion. I made rest a real priority during this early stage (although, to be honest, I was too unwell to exercise anyway).

My only activity during this phase was walking around the house and, on rare occasions, walking towards the end of my street and back. After nearly two months of sheer resting up, I started to feel that my energy levels were coming back.

I returned to my studies at university and naively believed that I could return to my exercise routine, too. This involved walking 2 miles each day back and forth from uni lectures, as well as a high-intensity boxing class three times a week.

When Lauren told me about the boom-and-bust pattern, I could easily identify with it, as I was experiencing the effects of pushing past my energy envelope, which was often met with symptoms of post-exertional malaise. Each day, I would only stop myself when my body told me, via payback symptoms, that it couldn't carry on.

Working with Lauren to help decipher my baseline, I was able to pace my activity levels going forwards by applying the 75-per-cent rule, committing to doing less activity than I was used to so as to help recoup my energy. I would take the bus most days to lectures instead of walking (however, I could safely get away with the 1-mile walk back from class once a week).

I was able to maintain this level of activity for two weeks without having a crash in CFS symptoms. This meant that I could then grade up my activity levels using a patient and gentle approach. It took some getting used to, as I have an overachiever personality and am prone to pushing myself. Lauren advised me to increase my weekly activity levels by attempting to walk 1 mile to lectures and 1 mile home – again, just once a week – and that if I could achieve this for 2 weeks without experiencing PEM, I could then attempt to progress my activity levels to new heights, using the grading approach.

I am now at a place where I can go jogging and take part in weekly boxing classes (while still leaving room for restorative approaches like Pilates and yoga at least once a week), and PEM is much a thing of the past. I still take care not to overdo it with my activity levels because I see the value in time spent resting and relaxing, which is just as important as time invested in 'doing' (whether this is exercise or any other form of physical activity for that matter).

Navigating exercise in CFS is ultimately about being realistic and honest with where your body is at during your particular stage of recovery. Applying Lauren's tools of pacing and grading has been vital for me in supporting my health and recovery from CFS.

CHAPTER 17

Lifestyle III – Detoxification

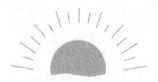

Only in the darkness can you see the stars.
Martin Luther King Jr, American Baptist and activist

The word 'detox' tends to get a bad rap, having become associated with all kinds of restrictive diets, supplements and health fads that promise transformed health, a boosted metabolism and weight loss, among other things. However, detoxification is a valid and vital weapon in your armoury when it comes to CFS and here's why.

The reality is that we live in a heavily polluted world, with chemicals everywhere – in our food, in the air we breathe, on our skin and so on. And although our bodies have their own in-built detoxification systems (the liver, kidneys, lymphatics, lungs, skin and gut), we are nevertheless overburdened with toxicity, which means that these systems are working overtime and often need some help. That's why it makes total sense for us to reduce the quantities of toxins that enter our bodies and support our detox systems, particularly if we have CFS. Because let's not forget that toxic chemicals (like heavy metals, moulds and pesticides from heavily sprayed fruits and vegetables) are very commonly associated with CFS, and one of the ways that they drive fatigue is through their ability to hinder the functioning of our mitochondria, immune system and hormones. They can also deplete essential nutrients and friendly gut bacteria and cause oxidative stress.

Detox 101

Here are some key strategies you can employ to support the detoxification process:

- **Antioxidant defence and the right foods to eat** Aim to supply your body with the nutrients it needs for detoxification to work at its very best. Antioxidant defence is essential in supporting detoxification. Opt for sulphur-rich foods, such as broccoli, garlic, onions, leeks and sprouts (provided you do not have a sulphur or FODMAP intolerance – see pp. 126–128). One of the most important antioxidants for neutralising free radicals is glutathione.

- **Establish regular toilet habits** If you do not urinate very frequently (sufficient hydration and drinking lots of water are key here) and if you struggle with constipation, these are some of the first things to address. Regularity is said to be having a bowel movement anywhere from three times a day to three times a week; however, you should be the judge of what is normal for you and whether you need to make yourself more regular.

- **Massage therapy** A trip to the spa may be just what the doctor ordered when you have CFS! Massage is great for the organs of detoxification, since it works by improving circulation, thereby supporting the liver and kidneys to perform their detoxifying functions, as well as promoting the drainage of lymph in the body. I recommend manual lymphatic drainage and deep-tissue massage, while general relaxation massages can also be supportive of the nervous system. These should always be carried out by a qualified therapist.

- **Dry skin brushing** This is an exfoliating body massage you can do at home to increase circulation and promote lymphatic drainage. Using a body brush, brush up towards the heart and chest, which is where the lymph system drains. Do this before a hot bath, as it can unclog the pores, ready for the body to sweat out toxins.

- **Sweat it out** I recommend hot baths and saunas (but do check with a healthcare professional first). Ten to fifteen minutes in a standard or far-infrared sauna, ideally three times a week would be a good way to go. And always remember to rehydrate afterwards.

Toxin alert

Here are some common toxins to watch out for:

- **Mercury** – found in silver amalgam dental fillings, large ocean fish (including swordfish and tuna), thermometers and light bulbs (broken), thimerosal (contained in some vaccines)

- **Lead** – found in old paints, pipes, petrol exhaust fumes, wicks in some candles (check labels or websites for information, wherever possible)

- **Aluminium** – found in deodorants, pots and pans, an adjuvant used in some vaccines, 'tin' foil, food and drink cans, takeaway containers, cosmetics

- **Mould** – found in homes (particularly older houses), in damp areas such as basements, ceilings and on the walls

- **Pesticides and antibiotics in the food supply:**
  - Over 1000 different pesticides are in use around the world. They are commonly used on crops, ending up as residues on our fruits and vegetables.
  - Antibiotic residues can be ingested by us when we consume conventional animal produce (which could be detrimental to the microbiome). There has also been a growing problem of antibiotic-resistant bacteria contaminating our meat and fish, causing food poisoning and making it difficult to treat infection.

- **Fluoride** – commonly used in the UK water supply and in dental products, such as toothpastes and mouth rinses

- **Chlorine** – found in swimming pools and added to tap water as a disinfectant

- **Toluene and benzene** – released when burning paraffin wax candles (**Note:** ARDERE candles avoid paraffin wax and are made from natural wax and lead-free wicks)

- **Triclosan** – a commonly used disinfectant found in antibacterial soaps, hand sanitisers, conditioners, body lotions and deodorants

- **Phthalates** – often called 'plasticisers', these are found in plastic wrappings such as cling film, cosmetics and skincare products, soap, shampoo, hair spray, perfume, air freshener, household cleaning products, plastic food-storage containers, shower curtains, toys

- **Oxybenzone** – found in conventional sun creams

- **Bisphenol A (BPA)** – found in metal food can linings, plastic food-storage containers, paper receipts, plastic water bottles

- **Formaldehyde** – found in nail polish, glues, paints, aerosol sprays, tobacco smoke, dishwashing liquid and fabric softeners, pet products

- **Flame retardants** – in mattresses, curtains, carpets, upholstery, electrical appliances, laptops, TVs, phones

- **Electro-magnetic fields (EMFs)** – household electrical devices (including hairdryers, washing machines, vacuum cleaners), televisions, radios, wireless technology and routers (mobile phones, laptops, Bluetooth devices, wi-fi routers), X-rays

Reduce your toxic load

Clearly, many of the toxins listed above are in things we all come across or use daily, so how can we go about reducing our exposure to things that are so ubiquitous and, in some cases, essential to modern-day living?

- **Invest in clean drinking water.** The tap water you drink varies in purity based upon where you live. Since standard water filter jugs only get rid of some chemicals and not all (plus, they pose the problem of being made from plastic), a reverse-osmosis water-filtration system is a great choice and should provide you with the purest water for drinking and cooking. Glass water-jug filters or countertop stainless steel filters are more affordable options (although the glass jugs may not filter as many contaminants).

- **Ventilate your home.** As well as keeping windows and doors open in good weather, you may want to invest in an air purifier and dehumidifier. Purifiers are helpful for removing harmful particles in the air, such as viruses and bacteria, as well as allergens, such as dust and pollen, while dehumidifiers are good at removing moisture from the air, decreasing humidity levels and helping to prevent mould exposure. If you already have a mould problem, it may be necessary to have the area in question professionally treated.

- **Go organic and purchase good-quality fresh produce.** Organic food is simply food in its natural state without the excessive use of manmade chemicals or antibiotics (it's about working *with* nature, not against it). Organic farming standards promote animal welfare, help to sustain the environment and support our health in the process. Animals should be pasture-raised and grass-fed, rather than caged and grain-fed. As a minimum, I would recommend you always try to opt for organic meat and poultry, eggs, soy (no more than twice weekly, if you have thyroid dysfunction or iodine deficiency) and dairy. And always wash your fruit and vegetables in apple cider vinegar, even if they are organic, to remove any chemical residues. Pesticide Action Network UK

(PAN UK) provide a list of the highest pesticide-sprayed fruits and vegetables in the UK, called the Dirty Dozen. When it comes to fish, go for wild-caught (or otherwise organic farmed) and look for the Marine Stewardship Council (MSC) blue tick or the Aquaculture Stewardship Council (ASC) logo to ensure that fish have been caught using socially responsible and sustainable practices. Avoid fish that are high in heavy metals, such as swordfish, tuna and king mackerel.

Note: it's not always necessary to look for 'organic' on labels – if you opt for locally sourced produce, and chat with suppliers, you are likely to find that the farmers adhere to organic farming practices without necessarily going through the organic certification process. Choosing local is great for the environment and helps you to eat seasonally, offering better nutritional value in the process, too. You could also try purchasing a weekly organic fruit-and-veg box (see Resources, p. 308).

- **Avoid storing food in plastic.** Use glass, ceramic or stainless steel, if possible. Likewise, switch to greaseproof paper from aluminium foil. Always consider what you are storing your food in and avoid heating food in plastic (in takeaway containers, for example).

- **Go natural with personal-care and cleaning products.** It's not just about what you eat, when it comes to lowering your toxic load – it's also about what you breathe in and put on your skin. Consider making the switch to non-toxic candles, bath and skincare, deodorants, cosmetics and cleaning products (see ARDERE in Resources, p. 308). If you would like to find out more about the ingredients to avoid in personal-care products, see, Resources, p. 308.

- **Consider biological dentistry.** A biological dentist believes that your oral health is connected to your overall health and wellbeing. Alongside the digestive tract, your mouth is connected to your immune and lymphatic systems, among others. One of the most common causes of heavy-metal toxicity is exposure to mercury amalgam fillings. If you suspect that you have had exposure to mercury from dental amalgam, a biological dentist can remove a metal filling safely from your mouth without the unwanted risk of exposing you to the mercury vapours and will use a much safer material for the filling instead. (For mercury-free dentistry in the UK, see Resources, p. 308.)

- **Turn off your wi-fi router before bedtime.** Turning off your wi-fi before bed reduces your exposure to EMF radiation when you are asleep. Switching your phone on to aeroplane mode also does this.

- **Keep your phone away from your body.** Keeping your phone on hands-free, rather than holding it close to your head, is another way to reduce EMF exposure.

Coriander tea decoction

Try my tea decoction – it is great for supporting the kidneys and clearing heavy metals. Drink it hot or cold throughout the day.

20g fresh coriander leaves
15g coriander seeds
5g fennel seeds (optional)
1 litre water

- Add the herbs and water to a saucepan and bring to the boil.
- Simmer over a medium–low heat for 30 minutes. If the mixture starts to reduce by more than half, add another 250ml water.
- Strain and decant into a glass jug and refrigerate overnight. It should keep for about a week in the fridge.

CHAPTER 18

Lifestyle IV –
Sleep and Stress

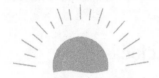

*The best bridge between despair and hope
is a good night's sleep.*
**E. Joseph Cossman, American inventor,
businessman, entrepreneur and author**

Sleep is the elixir of life. It helps us to calibrate emotions, fine-tunes our hormones (including the adrenals) and metabolism, curbs our appetites and restocks the immune system. In addition, our glymphatic system, which cleanses toxins from the brain, gets to work when we sleep.

It's common for those with CFS to experience trouble with sleep. They might feel that they are sleeping too much (common in the crash stage), not enough, despite high fatigue levels (common in the wired-and-tired stage) or that sleep is not restorative.

The architecture of sleep

Good-quality sleep is essential for supporting recovery and it is important to establish a regular sleep routine to facilitate this. There are two types of sleep: non-rapid eye-movement (NREM) and rapid eye-movement (REM). Most of our sleep is of the NREM type. REM is a stage where, as the name suggests, your eyes move from side to side very quickly, brain activity is heightened and you are more prone to vivid dreams. Some experts believe that REM sleep is when the memory gets a reboot, so that we can think more clearly.

Sleep is said to be broken up into stages and cycles – for example, three stages of non-REM sleep followed by one stage of REM. The final stage of non-REM is deep sleep. Each time you sleep you can have up to four cycles of this non-REM and REM sleep. During the deepest parts, the immune system is bolstered, tissues are repaired and the body is refreshed. A lack of deep sleep has been shown to contribute to a weakened immune system, as well as type-2 diabetes, obesity and heart disease.

Our biological clocks

Our sleep–wake cycles are regulated by something called a circadian rhythm, which is the body's twenty-four-hour internal clock that is regulated by light and darkness. Two of the main hormones involved in sleep that follow a circadian rhythm are melatonin and cortisol. Melatonin starts to peak at night, prompted by darkness, and is inhibited by light, so naturally starts to decline in the morning, particularly when we go outside. Then we have cortisol, which gets us bright-eyed and alert in the morning. So as melatonin wanes, cortisol gets us going to start a new day.

Of course, with CFS we tend to see a dysregulation in cortisol, to the extent that I have seen clients who have had low cortisol in the morning and high levels at night. Plus, when you are in the throes of the illness you might be spending less time outside, meaning less exposure to natural light, which interferes with the natural rhythm of melatonin. This is another contributing factor towards feeling sleepy during the day.

Discover your chronotype

Your chronotype is your body's natural inclination to go to sleep and wake up based upon times of the day (it is like the personality of your circadian rhythm). You might have heard people say that they are 'a morning lark' or 'a night owl', when referring to the times they get up and go to sleep. This is influenced by genetics; however, it can change as you age, too. When you know your chronotype, this can help you to make sense of your sleep preferences and how to align them with your daily activities. You can complete an online quiz to find out your chronotype (see Resources, p. 308).

What happens if you sleep too much?

Sleeping too much is likely to occur during the crash stage of the illness, and it is not uncommon for clients of mine to report sleeping for up to fifteen hours and still feeling exhausted when they wake up. While sleep is somewhat essential during the early stages of CFS (or during an exacerbation or PEM, especially if there is an infection to fight), a lot of my clients don't always realise that sleeping too much as time goes by can contribute to:

- the body becoming used to higher levels of sleep and later waking times
- the body feeling it needs even *more* sleep
- poor motivation, concentration and energy when awake.

So how do you know if you are sleeping too much? And how do you train your body to require less sleep?

First, you need to establish how much sleep you are getting over a twenty-four-hour period. If you find that you are sleeping for twelve hours or more, this might be too much. That said, there is no magic number or optimum amount of sleep you should be getting, as it varies for us all as individuals. Really, the problem is when the amount of sleep you are getting causes an *increase* in your fatigue levels.

If you are worried about sleeping too much, try keeping a sleep diary in which you jot down the following:

- how many hours you sleep each night
- how long it takes you to fall asleep
- what time you wake up each day
- whether you nap during the day and for how long

- anything else that you feel is relevant for you to build an understanding about your sleep.

One of the best solutions to sleeping too much is to establish regularity and a routine. Aim to get up at the same time each morning and begin to unwind, following your sleep-hygiene routines (see the next page), at the same time each night.

If you find that you are getting most of your sleep during the daytime – for example, you are sleeping between 5am and 2pm – start by adjusting the time that you wake up by setting an alarm, gradually moving it back thirty minutes at a time each day (in this case, start getting up at 1.30pm). This should mean that you start to feel tired earlier and therefore go to bed earlier (say, at 4.30am). Continue this process until you are going to sleep and waking up at the times you want.

Improving your sleep

One of the key reasons for not sleeping enough is because the nervous system is in fight or flight (see p. 46), due to a dysregulated pattern of cortisol, which, as we know, should be lowest at night because this is when we are meant to sleep. Not sleeping enough might also be a result of:

- finding it difficult to get to sleep at night
- broken sleep (i.e. waking multiple times during the night)
- waking very early, still experiencing high levels of fatigue
- going to bed very late.

The key to a good night's sleep involves:

- a calm mind
- regulated body temperature
- an empty bladder
- balanced blood-sugar levels.

 I often talk to my clients about sleep hygiene, which is all about incorporating lifestyle habits that may benefit sleep.

My top twelve sleep-hygiene tips

1. **Keep a routine.** Try to go to bed when you are sleepy and wake up at the same time every day. This is because your body likes routine and responds well to habit.

2. **Create a sleep-supportive environment.** Keep your bedroom cool (around 18°C) and ensure that your room is free of loud noises and harsh bright lights. You may want to consider blackout curtains, an eye mask or ear plugs, if necessary, and make sure that your mattress and pillow are comfortable and suit your sleep-position preference.

3. **Start to unwind one hour before bedtime.** Perform a sleep ritual that helps you to mentally prepare for sleep by setting the intention to relax and unwind an hour before bedtime. You might try a short breathing exercise (see p. 255), a meditation to relax the mind (see p. 255), listening to some calming music, some light reading or doing some mild stretching to relax the muscles.

4. **Avoid large meals two hours before bed.** This is because the digestive system will continue working and sleep may be disrupted (even if you do not wake up during this period). If you feel hungry before bed eat a light snack, such as a banana or a small handful of nuts, forty-five minutes before you go to sleep.

5. **Unplug.** We have analogue bodies trying to live a digital life, so to get a good night's slumber steer clear of technology an hour before hitting the sack. This one can be tough, but it's important. Technology can act as a stimulant, plus the blue light that is emitted from these devices can inhibit the release of melatonin. Switch to the 'night-shift' light mode on your devices in the evening or wear some blue-light-blocking glasses to avoid exposure.

6. **Avoid nicotine and alcohol.** Certain substances can impact the quality of our sleep, which means we spend less time in deep sleep,

making us more tired the next day. Alcohol, for example, can disrupt the stage of sleep most associated with repairing damaged cells, restoring brain function and renewing energy within the body.

7. **If you cannot sleep, get up.** This will help your brain to reassociate bed with rest rather than wakefulness – so instead of tossing and turning, get up and try to do something restful in another room, such as light reading or stretching. Once you feel sleep coming on again, return to bed. Also, don't look at the clock!

8. **Avoid heavy exercise before bed.** If you are at the stage of recovery where exercise is starting to become a part of your routine, avoid any strenuous exercise up to three hours before bed as this can spike cortisol levels (which should be lowest at night), making it hard to fall asleep. Yoga and Pilates are more restorative options to try instead.

9. **Don't drink too much fluid an hour before bed.** You don't want to be running to the bathroom in the middle of the night, so drink water during the daytime and only take small sips an hour before bed if you are thirsty.

10. **Use essential oils.** Aromatherapy is an excellent way to support good-quality sleep; many essential oils have a calming effect and sleep-promoting properties. It can also be beneficial to take a hot bath in the hours before bedtime. At ARDERE, we've developed a relaxing Epsom and Dead Sea salt bath blend full of muscle-easing magnesium, arnica and relaxing essential oils to help induce sleep; or you can try lighting a natural scented aromatherapy candle an hour before bed as part of your bedtime ritual, too (see Resources, p. 308).

11. **Write a list of what's on your mind.** Mind chatter and rumination can make it difficult to get to sleep, especially at times when anxiety is high. Write a list of your problems on a piece of paper and revisit them the next day, when you can think more clearly about solutions.

12. **Get outside into the sunlight (even in cloud cover).** This will help to establish a healthy cortisol and melatonin rhythm, anchoring your sleep–wake cycle. Anywhere from ten minutes should do the trick.

Daytime napping

In CFS, it's common for sleep cycles to become disrupted and to have to rely on sleeping during the day to get by. Many CFS patients take naps because their fatigue or brain fog symptoms are too strong during the day, or it may be a way for them to recover from PEM or an exacerbation in their symptoms.

I find naps to be restorative for CFS patients, if applied appropriately. It's all about experimenting with what works best for you and considering naps in the context of how they make you feel (i.e. what is the *purpose* of the naps?), based on their length, frequency and the time of day that you take them, as well as how well you are sleeping at night.

For example, if you find that daytime napping makes it harder to fall asleep at night, try avoiding them at least six hours before you normally go to bed. Naps that are longer than thirty minutes may increase the risk of grogginess, so try to keep them shorter than this to lower your risk of feeling unmotivated afterwards. If you are requiring multiple daytime naps, try to gradually reduce the number that you take over time, perhaps down to just one nap, which will support your circadian rhythm.

Also, what is your attitude towards taking a nap? Never associate yourself as lazy for wanting or needing one. If anything, you should retrain your brain to associate naps with being a pathway to productivity and recovery, as otherwise you could spend the rest of the day with low energy, whereas a nap could give you the refresher that you need to get through the day. Remember, the Spanish thrive off an afternoon siesta!

Stress

Every single one of us experiences stress in life. In fact, a report has revealed that more than 68 million GP visits in the UK in 2019 were related to stress.[14] Nevertheless, it's important to understand that stress can be a big driver in CFS specifically, and restoring balance in the nervous system is key to recovery.

As we saw on p. 48, sympathetic-nervous-system (SNS) activation can drive a lot of the symptoms we see in CFS. When the body is in a constant state of high alert, all energy drains from the body. Survival is the main priority and other bodily processes – such as our immune function or digesting the last meal we've eaten – are put on the back burner. Fight or flight is not an ideal state to spend most of your time in!

When I ask my clients about stress, some say they don't necessarily feel stressed, although it is clear that some stress is going on in the body (whether physical, mental or both). So many of us need to get off the crazy treadmill that is life in the twenty-first century. But how? Well, it's all about getting the body into a healing state, which involves calming down and balancing stress hormones, as well as activating the parasympathetic nervous system (PNS).

Top tips for dealing with stress

- Don't try to be perfect.
- Avoid people-pleasing.
- Be ok with leaving things undone that 'ought to be' done.
- Learn to say no.
- Schedule time for you, and only you.
- Switch off regularly and do nothing (that means absolutely nothing).
- Give yourself permission to do all the above (i.e. banish the guilt).

Adopt a mindful approach

Mindfulness is the art of being in the present moment, with a view to becoming more aware of your behaviours, thoughts, attitudes and bodily sensations to gain a better grasp on your lifestyle. It is a practice that involves observation without judgement and has been shown to significantly reduce stress and arouse feelings of calm and peace when practised on a regular basis.

Many of us can gravitate towards negative thinking, particularly when it is self-critical or self-destructive. With mindfulness, you simply notice a negative thought or observation as it pops into your head, then bring yourself back to the present moment and become aware, without trying to judge it. See your thoughts as clouds, observing them as they pass through your mind, rather than trying to focus on what they are trying to tell you. The mind is a bit like a monkey and is prone to wandering, but the trick here is not to beat yourself up when thoughts do arise; instead, try to gain a healthy sense of perspective on them by returning to the present moment and whatever you are focusing your attention on (whether the breath, chanting or a body scan). If you're interested in learning more about mindfulness practice, see Resources, p. 308.

Another great way to incorporate more mindfulness into your life is through meditation.

What is meditation?

Meditation is a relaxation practice that involves focusing your mind on a specific thing, while tuning out everything else around you. You might focus on the breath, a chant or parts of your body. Meditation is much more about the journey than the destination, and it helps to offset the negative effects of the bad or difficult days with CFS.

There are some really useful free apps that offer a variety of meditations you can try to suit your preferences (see Resources, p. 308).

Breathwork

A great way of reducing stress is through breathwork.

In our society, people continuously overbreathe. This includes lots of mouth breathing, upper-chest breathing and heavy sighing.

Although mouth breathing isn't always a bad thing, I recommend focusing on nasal breathing, which can enhance oxygen uptake and increase the production of nitric oxide, which facilitates oxygen transport around the body. Nasal breathing can also stimulate the vagus nerve, which controls parasympathetic activity in the body (it is a nervous-system tonic that activates the brakes on our stress response).

A well-known nasal breathing technique is alternate-nostril breathing, which involves inhaling and exhaling through alternate nostrils, one side at a time, to enable you to breathe more calmly and deeply.

Another great breathwork technique is the box-breathing method, where you inhale for four seconds, hold for four seconds, exhale for four seconds, hold again for four seconds and then repeat. This can help to reduce anxiety and improve mood and mental clarity.

For more on breathwork, see Resources, p. 308.

Get out into nature

Being in nature is highly beneficial for our health. We can gain benefits from sunlight, not only through the vitamin D our skin produces via sun exposure, but also because it helps to anchor our circadian rhythm. Sunlight also supports normal brain function and even helps us to generate ATP, that energy molecule I often go on about (see p. 64).

When I was unwell, I *always* used to feel way better when I was in the sunshine. Allow yourself at least ten to twenty minutes of outdoor exposure daily without sunglasses (so that the sunlight your eyes are naturally exposed to can anchor your circadian rhythm). When it comes to vitamin D, aim to strike a balance between protecting your skin from burning in the sun and getting vitamin D from sunlight.

Another way to benefit from nature is by grounding. This means realigning your body's energy by connecting to the earth – for instance, walking barefoot on the grass, sand or mud – which is very restorative!

Then there is forest bathing, which is all about immersing yourself in nature and taking in the benefits of the trees and natural surroundings. It's also helpful to do this without being hooked up to a phone or other device, so that you can connect more with your thoughts and feelings and less with technology.

Hydrotherapy

Hydrotherapy dates back thousands of years and is the use of water as a therapy.

One hydrotherapy practice I like is contrast showers, which involve alternating between hot and cold water when showering. Cold-water exposure is a form of hormesis (a type of low-grade metabolic stress) that can help to reduce inflammation and oxidation and support lymphatic and immune health in the body. Start by gradually reducing a hot shower to cold and holding it there for one minute, then turning it back to hot again, building up each day until you can tolerate five minutes of cold-water exposure.

An alternative to cold-water immersion is cryotherapy, where individuals stand inside a tank in which they are exposed to cold, dry air.

SAVANNAH, AGED TWENTY-EIGHT

In hindsight, I wish I had appreciated how most facets of my life contributed to my illness and/or recovery. That is not to scaremonger at all, but it speaks to the benefits of a holistic approach.

I used to see my illness in isolation from my gut health, my stress levels, my career, my relationships, etc. I thought that if I focused on curing my symptoms, I would find recovery. However, during my journey it became abundantly clear that I couldn't reach recovery without thinking about adapting my whole lifestyle.

I had to better my relationship with food, to find ways to lower my stress from work, to set healthy boundaries with my loved ones about what I needed, and develop strategies to positively respond to my environment, all while balancing my symptoms. This was overwhelming at times, but it provided me with a fantastic opportunity to take ownership of these aspects of my life and recognise the power I had in this regard. I now feel in tune with how interconnected and symbiotic my illness is with the other pillars in my life, and this knowledge has been incredibly helpful for me in getting closer to recovery. Unfortunately, treating symptoms topically will only take you so far.

CHAPTER 19

Mindset

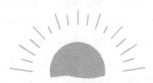

Acknowledging the good that you already have in your life is the foundation for all abundance.
Eckhart Tolle, spiritual teacher and author

Mindset plays a pivotal role in recovery from chronic illness. When you are unwell for a long period of time, your mental health is bound to be compromised. To recover, it is important to address the mental instabilities that have resulted from living with CFS and encourage a change in mindset.

Transforming your mindset is a key piece of the puzzle when it comes to overcoming CFS. Now, I am absolutely *not* saying that this illness is psychological. However, the point I want to make is that a physiological problem can be largely influenced by thoughts and our central stress response. The thoughts we think have a big influence on our symptoms and this is explained through the concept of psychoneuroendocrinoimmunology.

The mind-body connection

In the history of healthcare, the mind and body have been separated in silos. Nevertheless, science is now demonstrating just how interconnected the brain and body are, pointing towards an area of research called psychoneuroendocrinoimmunology (PNEI). Yep, it's a real mouthful, but it's quite simple if we break it down:

- Psycho = the mind and thoughts
- Neuro = the nervous system
- Endocrino = the endocrine system
- Immunology = the immune system

PNEI studies the relationship between the mind and these intricate body systems, and how if we have a particular thought this can influence our nervous and immune systems, as well as our hormones. Hence, every thought that you think influences your physiology in one way or another, for better or worse.

Anyone with a phobia will be able to attest to exactly how strong the mind–body connection is. Take somebody with arachnophobia. If you simply say the word spider, this will conjure up an image in that person's mind, causing their heart to race in fear, stirring up the fight-or-flight response. Another example is the urge to use the bathroom as you worry about an upcoming exam or interview, showing how nervousness can trigger physical symptoms.

What's more, did you know that you can increase stress hormones or mood-boosting chemicals, simply by thinking in a certain way? If you ruminate and catastrophise, you can increase cortisol levels, whereas if you engage in more positive and optimistic ways of thinking you can trigger the release of serotonin and dopamine (neurotransmitters that create a happy mood and feelings of wellbeing). So while you should never beat yourself up for feeling a little bit low now and again (it is perfectly normal and understandable when you are experiencing chronic illness), it is empowering to know that you are more in control of your health than you may have thought.

In essence, what we think, we *feel*!

CBT and CFS

Cognitive behavioural therapy (CBT) is a form of talking therapy that is used for a variety of health problems including IBS, depression, chronic pain (including fibromyalgia), eating disorders and, of course, CFS. It is based on the principle that you can support your health by changing the way that you think and behave. Therapists help you to spot and challenge unhelpful thought patterns, while encouraging more positive and helpful ones to take their place.

CBT can be a very helpful tool for people to gain more awareness of their mindset, while learning strategies to help overcome negative patterns of thinking (it is used within the NHS as a way of supporting CFS symptoms).

The ABCD model

Did you know that thoughts often stem from core beliefs?

The ABCD model takes the position that there is always an activating event (A), which results in a consequence (C). However, sitting in between lies a belief (B – an acceptance that something exists or is true, even if there is no proof), which we must dispute (D) and challenge to help create an effective new belief to deal more appropriately with the original activating event.

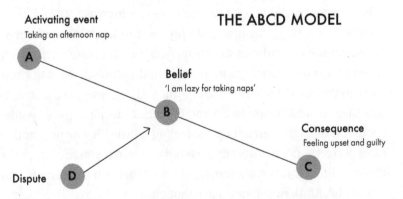

Take the example above. You decide to have an afternoon nap. The consequence is that you feel upset and guilty afterwards. And the reason for this is your belief that taking a nap means that you are lazy. How can you dispute this?

Ask yourself what would be more helpful to believe instead. Perhaps you could take the view that having a nap means you are honouring your body and listening to its needs? This way, you arrive at an effective new belief that will help to alleviate the negative states you were previously experiencing (more on 'states' on p. 264).

What are your beliefs about recovery?

Answer yes or no to these questions:

- Do you believe that recovery from CFS is possible?
- Do you believe that *you* can recover?

These are two very similar questions, but with different implications and meanings. The first asks you to look at your general views on recovery, whereas the second considers recovery within the context of your own case. If you answered no to the first question, then you likely answered no to the second. However, some people tell me that they believe others can recover from CFS, but that it is not possible for themselves. Why is this? Well, it is simply down to a belief system.

Common thought patterns to challenge in CFS

In CFS, it is common to experience the following unhelpful thought cycles (you may want to try the STOP process with these – see pp. 273–275):

- **Mental ping-pong** – where two different parts of your brain are batting against each other. For instance: I'm so tired. Maybe I should take a nap . . . but I always feel groggy after a nap. Maybe I should just push through . . . but then I'll just feel even worse . . .

- **Mind whizzing** – a form of mental noise, where thoughts are whizzing around your head like a blender. It's not so much the specific thoughts that are the problem here, but the speed at which you are experiencing them.

- **CFS goggles** – when you start to view the world through a chronic-illness lens, centred around the fear of increasing symptoms and leading to avoidance of activity. An example is hearing that a close friend has got engaged and that the wedding will be in Spain. Instead of being excited about the happy news, you put on your CFS goggles and worry, thinking: how am I going to make the flight? What if I can't get the food that I need over there? What if I crash? This level of worry exhausts your nervous system when you should be in the present moment with your friend, enjoying their happy news.

- **Snowballing** – when you wake up with a symptom and catastrophise the problem, saying the whole day is now 'ruined'.

- **Inner critic** – see p. 271.

Are you a perfectionist?

Perfectionism can be defined as setting extremely high standards (for yourself and others) and often results in negative consequences. In fact, it is a concept that does not quite match reality, as 'perfect' means different things to different people and so there can be no such thing.

On the surface, perfectionism is associated with achievement, a good work ethic and success, but deep down it can be a sign of insecurity and low self-esteem. It is like operating on a glass-half-empty, rather than half-full approach – and it's something I had to work on hugely in my recovery.

Perfectionist tendencies place a great deal of strain on the nervous system, which is why we must reprogramme these energetically expensive emotional ways of thinking, especially during recovery.

Consider how often you use language such as:

- 'I ought to . . .'
- 'I must . . .'
- 'I need to . . .'
- 'I should . . .'

Ultimately, dealing with perfectionism is about letting things –
the oughts, musts, needs and shoulds – go. Remember that your
worth is not based upon your accomplishments, and you are
valued and loved, regardless.

NLP and CFS

NLP (neuro-linguistic programming) and CBT are like two sides of the
same coin. They both help people to overcome limiting beliefs and move
towards a more positive way of thinking. However, NLP also offers a
model of how the mind perceives the information from the world
around us through our senses. Plus, it is content-free (which means
that you aren't required by the NLP practitioner to discuss your specific
concerns, since the tools you acquire can be applied at home, once you
have left your session).

I've been using NLP in my own private practice for some time now,
offering an NLP-mindset coaching course to support CFS clients, which
has contributed towards some incredible recoveries. Over the next few
pages, I will explore some key NLP principles that you can use to help
in your own recovery from CFS.

So what is NLP?
Let's start with a breakdown of the term neuro-linguistic programming:

- **Neuro:** refers to the nervous system, through which we gather
  information through our senses.
- **Linguistic:** refers to the language we use when we talk to ourselves
  (self-talk), as well as that used for communication between
  ourselves and others.
- **Programming:** the patterns that we adopt to utilise information
  gathered from our language and senses to improve our lives and
  achieve our goals.

NLP is a behavioural approach that studies the way our thoughts affect our state, providing a set of strategies to overcome negative states and reach our goals. It is a toolkit for dealing with life's opportunities and challenges and involves a number of language and behavioural techniques that can be learned, repeated and employed in daily life to change perceptions and behaviours.

What do we mean by 'a state'?

A state is the particular feeling that someone is in at any given time. For example, you might be lying in bed, relaxed or, alternatively, frustrated that you cannot fall asleep. The two states highlighted here are relaxed and frustrated.

One of my aims with clients is to help them break old patterns of behaviour and create new ones, while empowering them with more choice as to which states they create for themselves within a given situation. NLP shows us that states are fluid, and we have the power to change them to achieve our goals, using our knowledge and resources – but all too often we fail to see how we can utilise these in the right way, or we forget altogether that we have them.

The following are examples of states:

- Calm
- Relaxed
- Sad
- Hopeless
- Frustrated
- Motivated
- Angry
- Excited
- Anxious
- Optimistic
- Equanimous – calm, especially in a difficult situation

- Ambivalent – this can be a highly valued state (choosing not to get wrapped up in things that would normally affect you negatively)

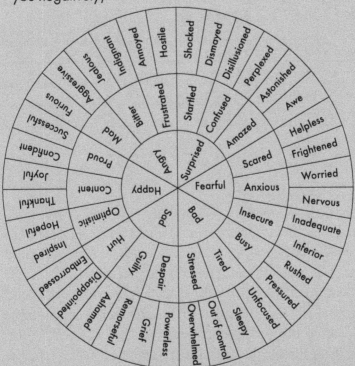

The wheel above can help you to develop your emotional intelligence and understand the variety of states that are possible for you to access.

What is the most useful state to be in?

The table on the next page highlights that someone performing heart surgery, for example, would not want to be in an anxious state when doing so.

Always ask yourself, what is the most appropriate state to be in for the task at hand? Asking this question brings an immediate insight into the most valued state to be in at that moment, helping you to direct yourself towards your goals.

Task	Least appropriate state	Most appropriate state
Performing heart surgery	Anxious	Calm, focused
Driving a car	Angry	Relaxed
Public speaking	Anxious	Calm, motivated
Running a marathon	Hopeless	Motivated
Doing an exam	Worried	Focused

When you have a thought, cells in your brain connect to send signals of information. This is called a neural pathway, and neural pathways are used for every thought that you think, as well as for performing habitual tasks, such as making a cup of tea or tying your shoelaces.

The more you think a particular thought, the stronger the signals in that pathway will be, firing information faster each time – as the saying goes, 'neurons that fire together, wire together'. Conversely, the less you use that pathway, the weaker it gets and the harder it is to use. An example is playing the piano. The more regularly you play, the easier it becomes and the better you get at it. If you don't practise for ten years, those neural connections will fade away and playing will become more difficult.

The same principle applies to negative thoughts. If you continue to repeat negative patterns of thinking, the brain makes it easier for you and it can fire those neural pathways very quickly. If you decide to think about something in a different way, however, your neural pathways will accordingly start to go in a different direction as it becomes more difficult for you to fire that 'negative' neural pathway. Put simply: use it or lose it.

This ability to make changes to the structure of your brain pathways is called neuroplasticity; simply put, the mind is malleable and you can therefore mould it – an idea that is very significant in the creation of habits and change. The practice of NLP is based on the concept of neuroplasticity, and it can help you to form new neural pathways to support health and happiness (it is also known as brain remapping).

You can visit my website for information on NLP courses (see Resources, p. 308).

NEUROPLASTICITY

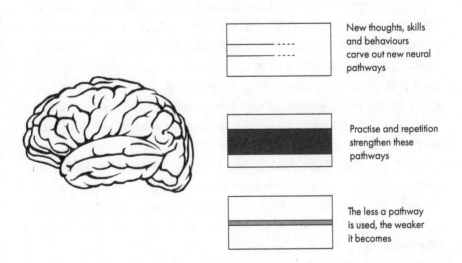

New thoughts, skills and behaviours carve out new neural pathways

Practise and repetition strengthen these pathways

The less a pathway is used, the weaker it becomes

When you end up in a vicious cycle of toxic thought patterns, this can often perpetuate or exacerbate symptoms due to the stress placed upon the nervous system. Often in CFS, you go through cycles of stress, worry or panic because of the symptoms themselves (fatigue or brain fog, for example). Learning to tap into the way that your mind has programmed itself over time can help you to make great progress in your recovery journey. It is very much like brain training; remember, the brain is like a muscle that you need to flex to make stronger. You just need to flex it in the right way to get the body into a healing state.

Some key NLP techniques include:

- language patterns and well-formed outcomes (WFOs)
- submodalities
- the STOP technique
- presuppositions.

Language patterns and well-formed outcomes (WFOs)
Did you know that the language you use can create a state? For example:

- I want you to NOT think about Marilyn Monroe riding a purple elephant for five seconds.

What happened? I'll bet you immediately thought of Marilyn Monroe riding a purple elephant! This is because the brain cannot directly process negatives such as, 'Don't think about X' without first understanding the instruction. And to understand the instruction, the brain must first process the idea of what (in this example) Marilyn Monroe and a purple elephant are, so that it can then *not* think about them. Thus, an instruction with a negative, known as a 'negative want', will always create the opposite of the desired effect.

A sentence like, 'I am *not* negative; I spend all my time making sure I am *not* stressed,' contains two negative wants. As a result, someone who says this will step into the state of being negative and stressed (the things they are actively trying to avoid), simply by virtue of the language they are using.

Our aim is to instil positive motivation, which is all about reaching goals, rather than negative motivation, which is more concerned with avoiding problems. To do this, try writing down three health goals you would like to achieve over the next year (see opposite). The one rule here is to make sure your goals are listed in positive terms (i.e. they are about what you *do* want, not what you *don't* want).

Examples:

- I want to have boundless energy.
- I want to have a healthy-functioning digestive system.
- I want to have great memory and concentration.
- I want to be more relaxed.
- I want to be resilient.

Health goal number 1	
Health goal number 2	
Health goal number 3	

Now, for each of these three goals, ask yourself:

- How will I be able to tell if I have achieved my goal? What will I see, feel, hear?
- Is this goal reasonable?
- What is the first step towards achieving this goal?
- Do I have the knowledge and/or resources to achieve this goal?
- How might I sabotage reaching this goal in the future?

In NLP, we call this exercise well-formed outcomes (WFOs), and it helps you to understand what your goals are, while examining the blocks that prevent you from reaching them.

AVOID HIDDEN NEGATIVES
Hidden negatives are words that easily trip us up into negative states. Here are some examples:

- **Managing** – 'I am managing my illness.' This implies that you've still got the illness and buys into the static nature of this thing that is still in existence. A positive reframe might be 'I am improving my health.'

- **Control** – 'I am controlling my symptoms.' A good word to go for instead would be 'choice', i.e. 'I am choosing to nurture my health.'

- **Freedom** – 'I want complete freedom from my symptoms.'
  Freedom can be a good thing, but here it is about the desire to be
  'free of' something.

- **Carefree** – this uses the word 'care', which means that you are
  stepping into the state that you seek to be 'free' from.

Submodalities

NLP also works by studying the structure of our subjective experience. It helps to examine the way that the brain and nervous system experience the world, using the power of language and our five sensory systems (sight, hearing, touch, smell and taste).

In fact, we use our senses to encode memory, thought and our way of seeing the world. For example, if you think of a slice of pizza, the chances are a picture of a slice of pizza will pop into your head. This would be a visual example of how we encode memory.

Our internal representations based on the five senses are called modalities, and we can chunk these down further into submodalities, which include the following:

- Colour
- Clarity
- Size
- Positioning
- Speed
- Volume

I like to call this the 'cinema of the mind'. If we can make changes to the cinema of the mind, or submodalities, we can make great changes in our lives, based on how we encode memories and thoughts, thus changing the meaning of an experience. Going back to the pizza – if the picture is colourful and up close, it might suggest that you really want and desire that pizza. However, if it is in black and white and positioned low down or behind you, this could indicate that the pizza has not much appeal for you at all.

The table opposite shows some examples of submodalities.

Sight	Sound	Touch
Black and white or colour	High- or low-pitched	Heavy or lightweight
Near or far	Fast or slow	Smooth or rough texture
Bright or dim	Clarity	Hot or cold temperature
Size of picture	Rhythm	Shape
Location	Verbal or tonal	Size
Movie or still-frame	Loud or quiet	Vibration
If it's a movie; is it fast, normal or slow?	Whose voice? One or many?	Pressure
Focused or unclear	Fading in and out?	Location
3D or flat	Other background sounds?	Large or small area
Associated versus disassociated	Mono or stereo	Constant or intermittent

Giving yourself a hard time – thinking things like, I should be improving much faster than this. Or, I'm not very good at applying these lifestyle changes. Or, Why am I so rubbish at everything? – is a sign that your inner critic is at work. Try shrinking down your critical self-talk and internal dialogue by imagining the stream of negativity being sung by a group of operatic sopranos, for example, or perhaps being played super fast on a tape, or sounding like a cartoon character, until all credibility is destroyed. You could also imagine the criticism in the voice of someone who loves you, which then makes it incongruous and more difficult for you to buy into that narrative. It shifts the emotional weight of your thoughts and therefore helps you to challenge and change them.

Try this: picture your wellbeing as a clearly focused, life-sized, realistic colour, 3D moving picture with sound and movement. Project this far into the future, so that you can help shape your system towards this way of being.

Play around with the submodalities of negative memories or thoughts:

- Shrink the image down.
- Send it to the other side of the world – to Australia, for example.
- Change the colour to black and white.
- Make the movie play on full speed or very slowly.
- Give it a Mickey Mouse voice.

ASSOCIATION AND DISASSOCIATION

Association and disassociation are two important submodalities that refer to how we see ourselves in our memories or thoughts.

Association is where you are fully and viscerally connected to an experience, so that it's like you are physically still there, in that moment, viewing it through your own eyes. This means that the emotions within that experience are somewhat intensified. By contrast, when you see yourself as a body playing out the memory, this shows that you are disassociated from the experience, which softens the emotional intensity.

I always advise my clients to try to associate with the good and disassociate from the bad memories. To associate, try to tap into the sensory experiences of the memory in question. If you are trying to associate with a memory of running and feeling energised, for example, focus on the colours and picturesque scenery around you, as though you are there right now – feel the breeze on your skin and hear the sound of your feet pounding the pavement. To disassociate, try to imagine that you are sitting in the projector room of a cinema, viewing yourself down in the audience watching a movie of your memory play out on the cinema screen. This helps to put distance between you and the memory in question.

Anchoring

Anchoring is the process of associating a stimulus with an internal state, so that the state can be reaccessed quickly and easily via the stimulus. An example of a useful anchor is the smell of sun cream reminding you of a blissful, relaxing holiday.

Set up your own anchor

Can you think of a time when you felt really good about yourself? Close your eyes and try to fully associate with that memory. Take a deep breath. Feel what you felt in that moment and let that feeling flood your entire body from the top of your head to the tips of your toes. When that state is at its peak, it is time to set up the anchor. Squeeze your thumb and forefinger together for five seconds as you continue to experience the positive state. You should now be able to access this state easily at any time you want by simply squeezing your thumb and forefinger together to create an association with it.

Note: it is also possible to set up anchors using colours, sounds or smells. For example, a blue pen might be your anchor for calm, a green plant for focus or a yellow sunflower for energy. A humming sound might be your anchor for relaxation, while you may associate a smell of lavender with peacefulness.

The STOP technique

The STOP technique is all about catching yourself during unhelpful moments. It relates to a state you do not want to be in. I call this the pothole, and it can involve unhelpful thought patterns and negative self-talk that do not serve you.

Here's how it works:

1. Notice when you are heading into a pothole.

2. Say the word 'STOP' in a firm but not chastising manner. At the same time, use both your hands to gesture a stop sign and step away from the spot that you are currently standing on. (**Note:** this technique works best by using sensory modalities, which is why moving your body around and saying the words aloud, rather than in your head, will initially be more powerful, helping to teach your neural pathways to go in a new direction.)

3. You now have a choice; to stay on the path that you are currently going down or to head into a new (more helpful) way of thinking. If you decide to opt for a new way of thinking, then step again, towards a new spot on the ground. You are now embodying your own inner coach who is supportive and empowering. Make a statement that empowers you. For example, 'Well done! You are on your way towards achieving your goals.' Then ask yourself, 'What do you want?'

4. Step into another spot and reply to your inner coach. State your goals in positives, such as, 'I want to believe that recovery is possible' (rather than 'I don't want to feel hopeless about my illness').

5. Step back on to the coach spot, and in coach mode ask, 'And how are you going to achieve that?'

6. Returning to the previous spot, consider the state required to achieve your goal – say, empowerment – and use a memory or experience to create an anchor to associate with it. Now take yourself back to a time where you have previously experienced that state – seeing what you saw, feeling what you felt and hearing what you heard. If you can't think of one, you can borrow from someone you know, a TV character or an object that has similar qualities to those you want to access. Or try using an analogy (for example, 'I want to feel empowered like my dad, when he set up his own business') or a simile ('I want to feel as energetic as the warm, bright yellow sun' or '. . . as brave as a lion'). Now close your eyes, breathe into that state and allow it to fully permeate your

body. Let the colours that you associate with that state fully flood you like a ray of light.

Note: if you are struggling to access a state, make sure you are fully 'in' the movie of your mind (associated) and not just watching it (disassociated). Focus on your feet and ground yourself. This is about visualisation and using the power of your imagination.

7. Channel that state into the present moment and flash it forwards into the next few hours, days and weeks, helping you to achieve whatever goal you want.

The STOP process is particularly helpful when experiencing any unhelpful thoughts. Repetition of this technique is what makes all the difference. Remember it is not just about appearing calmer or optimistic about recovery; it is about feeling happy, confident, empowered and joyful, too. There are so many wonderful states available to access.

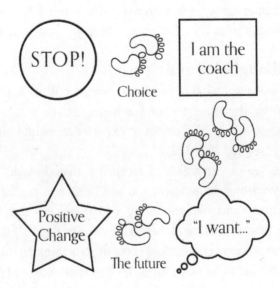

Presuppositions

In NLP, there are some common principles known as presuppositions that we can apply to help us look at the world, and get ourselves out of sticky situations:

- Behind every human behaviour is a positive intention.
- The person with the best flexibility exerts the most influence in any given situation (it's about bending with the wind!).
- There is no failure, only feedback. Every experience can be viewed as an opportunity to learn.
- It is not what happens to you, but what you *do* with what happens to you that makes all the difference.
- You cannot fail to communicate. You can only choose to do so unconsciously or consciously. For example, if John walks into a room saying nothing, he is still communicating something (through his body language), whether he is aware of this or not.
- If you aren't getting the response you want, do something different.

Other positive-mindset approaches

There are numerous ways in which a positive mindset can be helpful when recovering from CFS. Let's take a look at some of them.

Keep a thought journal

When you wake up, what is your first thought? What is your internal dialogue? What thought cycles do you have going on in relation to your illness? Do you wear CFS goggles or experience mental ping-pong or snowballing (see pp. 261–262)?

Often, we see our thoughts as facts, but that does not mean that they are. By writing them down, you will be able to put some distance between yourself and your thoughts, so that you can start to see how unhelpful or inaccurate some of them truly are. Try regularly documenting your thoughts to uncover any blind spots in your thinking. Can you start to see how they are influencing states, bodily experiences and symptoms?

Opposite is an example thought journal (and a template for you to fill in):

Date	Situation What were you doing?	Emotion(s) What did you feel? How strong was this feeling (out of 10)?	Automatic thoughts What were your thoughts? How much did you believe each of them (out of 10)?
Monday	I was at a restaurant, waiting for my meal to arrive.	Anxious 9/10	This food is going to make me crash; I just know it. I'm going to wake up tomorrow so bloated. 10/10
Thursday	I had an argument with my partner.	Angry 7/10	Why does he always have to be so unreasonable? I'm sick of being treated like this. 8/10
Friday	I woke up and some symptoms had returned (fatigue, brain fog).	Worried 9/10 Frustrated 8/10 Guilty 10/10 Hopeless 10/10	It's getting worse, I know it. It's because I overexerted myself last night. I don't think my health will ever return. 10/10

Date	Situation What were you doing?	Emotion(s) What did you feel? How strong was this feeling out of 10?	Automatic thoughts What were your thoughts? How much did you believe each of them out of 10?

Some useful questions to ask yourself when journaling:

- Am I comparing what is happening to me now with the past?
- Am I thinking about the future based on how I feel right now?
- How do I compare myself with others?
- How do I see myself?

The rest of what you write in your thought journal can be simply an unstructured stream of consciousness on your daily thought cycles. Just write whatever comes to you in the moment.

Keep your thought journal with you as much as possible over the next few weeks and keep coming back to it for reflection. Ask yourself: am I confusing thoughts with facts?

Top tip: labelling negative thoughts in your journal as ANTs (automatic negative thoughts) helps you to detach yourself from this way of thinking. Then look for evidence against any ANTs to help you develop alternative and more helpful thoughts. You could use the ABCD model (see p. 260) to help with this.

Become a narrator of your environment

Here is a useful tool for stepping out of your head (especially when you are 'mind whizzing') and into the present moment, releasing stress hormones from your system. You can do this anywhere – on a bus, a train or even while walking.

- Simply observe your environment and, in your head, state three things that you see around you. For example: baby in a pram, lady in a red coat, dog licking its paws.
- Now state three things that you can feel, and three that you can hear.
- Observe and breathe into the sensory experiences around you.

The trick is to avoid analysing or telling stories off the back of your observations (for example, I don't like the way that lady is looking at me; or, Did I feed the dog before I left the house?). Analysing engages your left (thinking) brain, instead of your right (feeling) brain. Simply observe your thoughts and don't try to make sense of them.

The more you practise this, the easier it gets. After five minutes, you will access a state of relaxation and become more present.

Deal with anxiety

Anxiety is a feeling of fear or apprehension about the future and is your body's natural response to stress. It is there to help you in certain instances, but if it is ongoing it can be a real hindrance. If you regularly worry about CFS symptoms, for example, dealing with this anxiety can be very important in helping to reduce the stress load on your body.

Think of anxiety as a guard dog in your home that thinks it is helping, even though it is biting the leg of the friendly postman or the neighbour. Often, anxiety causes us to react to perceived rather than actual threats, and recognising this is important. Try telling yourself, Thanks, but you are not needed right now; or, Thank you, mind.

Affirmations

Affirmations are positive statements that allow you to overcome unhelpful self-talk and guide you on a path towards self-love and acceptance.

Try saying three affirmations in the mirror each day, even if you don't believe them initially. The more you practise them, the more your subconscious will start to accept them into your reality – for example:

- 'I am healthy.'
- 'I am strong.'
- 'I am resilient.'
- 'My body does amazing things for me each day.'

Practise gratitude

Gratitude is being thankful for all that we have in our lives. It is impossible to feel sad and grateful at the same time, which is why gratitude can shift us into a new, positive perspective where we can see the good things in our lives. In difficult times, it can often feel hard to find things to be grateful for, but really there is always something. It can be as simple as the following:

- 'I am grateful to have a roof over my head.'
- 'I am grateful that I had the energy for a short walk today and was able to enjoy the sunshine.'
- 'I am grateful to have supportive people in my life.'
- 'I am grateful to have slept well through the night.'
- 'I am grateful for the progress I have made in my health journey.'
- 'I am grateful for all the lessons I have learned because of my illness.'

Try to find three things you are grateful for each day, no matter how small they may be.

Healing your trauma

Working through any trauma or ACEs (adverse childhood experiences – see p. 84) that you have experienced is a really important facet in CFS recovery, and key for benefiting the health of your brain and nervous system. What's more, many people are traumatised by the illness in and of itself.

A lot of my clients describe themselves as highly sensitive people, meaning that they are sensitive to their environments, lifestyle and, of course, life events. It is important to seek out professional support (say, from a psychologist) if you are dealing with trauma of any kind, but there are also a variety of self-help tools that you can access at home.

Practise the emotional-freedom technique (EFT)

One strategy that can really benefit trauma is EFT. This combines ancient Chinese acupressure (described as acupuncture without the needles – performed on specific points of the body) with modern psychology. It involves tapping on multiple points in the body, while you focus on a specific problem or emotion, acknowledging it by saying reassuring words to yourself as you release negative or distressing emotions. This could be something like, 'Even though I am feeling exhausted, I deeply and completely accept myself'; or, 'Even though I feel worthless and unproductive, I deeply and lovingly accept myself.'

The specific places to tap on are the endpoints of the body's major meridians (believed to be channels of subtle energy that flow through the body, see diagram below).

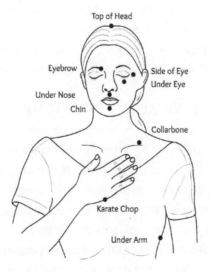

EFT can be used for anxiety, fatigue, stress, pain and limiting beliefs, as well as for supporting relationships. It works by sending calming signals to the amygdala in the brain (where the fight-or-flight mechanism originates), allowing it to calm down and process and release emotions.

To find out more about EFT (also known as 'tapping'), see Resources, p. 308.

GRACE, AGED THIRTY-TWO

As a chronic overachiever and perfectionist with a busy mind and tough inner critic, my thoughts, self-talk and emotional states were important to understand, soothe and address, as I was often operating in fight-or-flight mode, which wasn't a state in which healing could happen. In fact, I'd go as far as to say that I no longer knew how to rest – my nervous system had become overwhelmed after I got EBV [Epstein–Barr virus] and never recovered, becoming hard-wired to operating in the sympathetic nervous system. Through Lauren's NLP course, and particularly through journaling, I realised that a big part of my exhaustion was being exacerbated by mental and emotional exertion. NLP has given me some powerful tools to soothe and support my mind and emotional states. My mind and body are now working more in harmony, rather than against one another and out of sync. As a result, I move through the world very differently and am able not only to support my recovery from CFS symptoms, but also to handle the demands and strains of work and life more generally, too. Over time, this has contributed to the calming and steadying of my nervous system and wellbeing overall.

STEVE, AGED FIFTY-EIGHT

To be honest, learning to develop a positive mindset in the midst of having your life turned upside down by a chronic illness is not an easy thing. It takes time. It takes practice. But by embracing tools such as meditation, NLP and EFT, as well as getting out into nature, listening to music – whatever it is that brings out happiness and positivity in your soul – you will begin to climb back and find a sense of worth that CFS has stripped you of. On your recovery journey, you will have great days, you'll have low days and then you'll have days when you just want to give up on the whole thing. Adopting the mindset that 'this is normal', that 'it's part of the process', will help you to find your way back. Oh, and I'd really recommend finding some 'recovery buddies' on social media or at a local support group who are going through the same experiences as you. Having those friends will really help you to have clarity of mind when life gets challenging.

Social Media and CFS

Social media can often be a blessing and a curse, both generally speaking and, more specifically, when recovering from CFS.

A lot of vulnerable people turn to social media when they are dealing with poor health, putting themselves out there to gain support and find a way to voice their own struggles, while perhaps hoping to help others going through similar things too. However, some may share only the best of their recoveries and not the hardships or instabilities. As such, the internet can become a place that breeds comparison, fear and worry in people that they are not 'doing it right'.

There can be real danger in following advice from unqualified social media accounts and bloggers, which, while often well meaning, may not always have the most accurate or evidence-based information.

Another thing I would say about social media is that we often tend to doom-scroll – looking at negative news stories and using social media as a way to screen for fear-triggering information – and this can apply to recovery and whether it is (or isn't) possible with CFS. Avoid doom-scrolling at all costs, and try to take social media with a pinch of salt. Remember that it is an edited version of reality, and that you need to surround yourself with a positive and optimistic community of CFS warriors who can attest to the fact that recovery is indeed a possibility.

Also, avoid comparing your journey with that of others. Stay in your own lane!

Recovery is not a race

Recovery is not a race, and you don't have to feel guilty if it takes longer than you thought it would.

I do not kid anybody who comes to see me in clinic into thinking that working with me is going to be a quick process. If you want to make long-term changes to your health and wellness, it is most definitely going to take time. Remember to focus always on how far you have come (small steps most definitely count) and try to understand what the experience has taught you overall.

If you are still on your journey, do not be alarmed when you experience minor glitches here and there. You have to be prepared for these, so arm yourself with the following:

- **Patience:** be patient, and avoid worrying about the time it is taking to reach your health goals.

- **Kindness:** be kind to your body, and listen to it, as it is always communicating with you. A loving relationship towards yourself is almost always going to facilitate healing.

- **Understanding:** understand the process. Chronic illness is not like coming down with the flu and then bouncing back within a week. You need to understand the nature of what you are dealing with, and that long-term measures need to be put in place as a response.

Practise regular self-care

Self-care is any deliberate practice that you undertake to benefit your mental, physical or emotional health. It is all about paying attention to *you* – not in a narcissistic way, but in a loving way.

Here are some examples of self-care:

- Taking a relaxing Epsom salt hot bath (see ARDERE in Resources, p. 308)
- Lighting a scented candle (see ARDERE in Resources, p. 308)
- Applying a face mask or scrub (see ARDERE in Resources, p. 308)
- Using a hot-water bottle (see ARDERE in Resources, p. 308)
- Meditation or yoga
- Going for a walk
- Cooking a healthy meal (see ARDERE in Resources, p. 308)
- Repeating a positive mantra to yourself in the mirror (for example, 'I am well')
- Practising daily gratitude or journaling

All these acts and many more can contribute to filling up your cup and building a positive relationship with yourself. Incorporating practices such as these into your routine is a great way to counter the mental-health challenges that can come with chronic illness and help you to feel more resilient.

Top tip: always ask yourself, 'Am I in my head or in my body?' For those of you who are prone to anxiety, you may be more likely to be listening to the stories in your head, instead of any physical signs and symptoms or sensations. Once you spot this, draw your energy back inwards, towards your centre, and ground yourself. You can do this through a gentle internal body scan that ends by focusing on your feet on the ground, or through cradling yourself in a kind and loving self-hug.

CONCLUSION

Out of the Fog and Into the Light

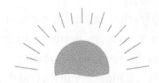

We so often expect there to be a transcendent light-bulb moment when we wake up one day and every symptom has gone. The reality, however, is that there isn't a finish line. It's simply about achieving a better level of physical functioning and understanding how to bypass the bottle-necks that are keeping you from moving forwards when you have a crash in symptoms.

So how do you know when you've recovered? It's the point when you realise you have spent more time in your day thinking about all the things you are doing and planning for the future, rather than living through the lens of your illness. (Remember: *illness does not define you.*) And it's when you find you have longer and longer periods without a crash, when you can start to function more optimally again.

Over time, with the help of the strategies in this book, your func-tional capacity should improve more and more. But it's not a fast track to perfect health. It's more of a fluid and non-linear approach towards improving your wellbeing and optimising your state of health, so that it is better than it was before – for which you will have a deep sense of gratitude. Plus, by sticking with the healthy-lifestyle pillars in Part 3, you can substantially reduce your risk of developing other chronic diseases, such as type-2 diabetes, obesity, heart disease and cancer, increasing your longevity and quality of life in the long run.

CFS is not only physically and psychologically exhausting, but also incredibly confusing, not knowing how your health is going to be each day when you wake up and feeling like one thing hits you after the other. It is difficult socially, too, because you become compartmentalised as a hypochondriac when this is just not the case. I wanted more than anything to be healthy, but each day I battled symptoms that knocked me down, despite my best efforts to get well and lead a normal life.

Research – hope for the future

There are so many people out there in the dark suffering with CFS, who don't have the necessary support network to understand or provide treatment protocols to help them, or who lack the financial resources to look into alternatives. It is a highly controversial medical issue, but this is not a reason for professionals not to take it seriously.

There is a long way to go in CFS research and, while functional medicine, looking at gut health, dietary adjustments and lifestyle interventions absolutely helped me in many ways, I fundamentally believe that more funding needs to go into orthodox medical research of this complex condition in order to formulate future treatments.

A UK study has revealed that over a period of 9 years, only £10 million was spent in the UK researching CFS, which works out at £40 per patient. In comparison, rheumatoid-arthritis research added up to £320, epilepsy research £200 and multiple sclerosis £800 per patient.[15]

Here's what we need for better CFS research moving forwards:

* Much larger studies involving more participants
* Identification of subgroups – there is a general view that there may be subgroups of patients with slightly different symptoms and underlying pathophysiologies
* Collaboration among researchers to see the bigger picture – for example, immunologists need to work with gastroenterologists and neurologists, etc.
* More funding

All that said, as scientific investigations continue, our grasp of how our complex systems speak to one another in this illness is widening. Hopefully, this will progress an understanding of how to establish appropriate diagnostic parameters, possible sub-types of the illness and, importantly, effective treatments.

My aim here is to reach as many people as possible who are going through a health battle like the one I did.

Never feel alone on your journey. Allow this book to be your comfort – a guide to learning more about the functional approaches that have helped me to get to where I am today, with a full-time business and a thriving wellness clinic.

You have it in you to influence your health for the better. Let this book empower you as you do so.

APPENDICES

APPENDIX I

Troubleshooting

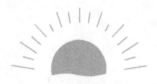

If you have read Part 3 and implemented some of the key strategies, but you don't feel you are getting the results you would like, here's a brief guide to some key factors that may be impeding your recovery progress.

Dealing with overwhelm

Take a deep breath. The concept of recovery can often be overwhelming.

Be kind to yourself and accept that there is no magic formula for recovery. Step away from these feelings and try to centre yourself with some deep breathing. And remember that sometimes, doing less is better than trying a million things all at once. Start small, and don't bite off more than you can chew. Approach everything in bite-sized chunks and know that time is a great healer as well.

'I've tried everything!'

This is a big one that I hear all too often. You may think that you have tried every strategy on the planet, but the reality is that you probably haven't!

For example, you may have tried a nutritional change, such as going gluten-free, but not mastered the art of eating in a mindful state, which could be a gamechanger for your gut health and recovery.

Don't be disheartened – because every step you take brings you closer to finding your feet with it all. Don't ever let a lack of immediate results dissuade you from the efforts you are making. Patience is a key trick of the trade in CFS recovery, and you need to make firm friends with it.

Keep the faith to get back up again when it feels like you are getting knocked down. And remember that a particular approach may not have worked because it was not done at the right stage *for you* – it was not implemented at the appropriate stage of *your* recovery journey, for example – so don't be afraid to try it again.

Challenge your thinking when you start to question your progress if something isn't an instant fix. The reality is, every lifestyle change you make is an invaluable investment in moving you forward (even if you do not realise it) and can be a crucial stepping stone towards recovery.

'I'm never quite there yet'

If you are feeling despondent because you are not quite 'there yet', consider the progress you have already made on your recovery journey. This can help to reframe your experience, while focusing on all the positive things that your illness has taught you: the value of good health, the importance of lifestyle in preventing other illnesses and the other vital life lessons you have gained along the way.

Inspire yourself forwards but measure yourself backwards.

I like to say to my clients that this is a way of 'building the evidence' of recovery, and, once you can look back and prove to yourself that progress and recovery exist, there is no reason to say that more cannot be achieved in the future.

When scepticism gets in the way

We've all had trouble with our inner sceptics from time to time, and it goes without saying that this illness can have you surrounded by external sceptics, too, who may invalidate your experience. Push all that aside and be aware that recovery from this illness means suspending your disbelief. Build those neural pathways (see p. 266) towards an optimistic approach that focuses on the good and crowd out the negative, always.

Focus on the mini wins

Try to focus on the mini wins: those little golden moments when you realise how far you have come – say, that short jog you never thought you'd be able to do; or when you realise you can eat a food without your body throwing a hissy fit. Just because something seems to be a small feat, that does not mean it's not noteworthy. Celebrate those moments because they *matter*. *You* matter, and your health matters!

Dealing with crashes

In CFS, you must develop the ability to endure the emotional ups and downs of recovery, when it can often feel like a game of snakes and ladders. I call this the 'bounce back', and it refers to how well you deal with a crash and navigate your way forward to bounce back from them.

Ask yourself, how hardy is your mindset in dealing with crashes? Are you talking to yourself negatively and beating yourself up about your symptoms? Could you be kinder to yourself? Complete the checklist below to explore some of the barriers towards recovery.

	✔	X
I do not believe it is possible to recover.		
I'm constantly wondering about the cause of my symptoms.		
I will only ever be 'managing' my health and never be free of this illness.		
I blame myself for my illness.		
I constantly focus on my symptoms.		
I constantly filter for symptoms.		
I worry about crashing.		
I often put myself down.		
I don't have the resources to recover.		
I often feel overwhelmed.		
I constantly focus on what I need to do to recover.		
I often compare myself to others with CFS and think I am worse off.		
I often compare myself now to the 'me' before I got CFS.		

If you tick five or more of these boxes, it could be a sign that you have a few recovery blocks in your mind. For example, when you think that recovery is no longer possible, it often leads to giving up. Spotting this belief, dealing with any myths around it and reframing it are important, so that you can figure out how to get back on the horse.

It is important to understand that your life *will* look different from before because of your experience with CFS, but this needn't be a bad thing. In fact, some of the circumstances you were in before CFS might have made you more susceptible to illness, so trying to get back to the 'old' you may not be in your best interests. No one goes back to leading the exact same lifestyle they had before CFS – and that's ok!

APPENDIX II

Complementary Approaches to CFS

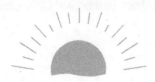

It is strongly advised that you always work with a trusted and experienced practitioner who has trained in the treatment in question.

We've talked about suspending disbelief, and you will no doubt have come across your fair share of CFS warriors visiting holistic therapists and exploring all kinds of what might, on the surface, seem like weird and wacky therapies to improve health outcomes, functionality and quality of life.

As long as these do no harm, I try to stay open-minded about complementary therapies in CFS recovery. In fact, I – and many of my clients – have experienced benefits from them, so let's explore some of them here.

The Perrin Technique

The Perrin Technique is an osteopathic approach that manually supports disorders affecting the nervous system, such as CFS and fibromyalgia.

Treatment involves weekly sessions where a form of massage called effleurage is performed on the back and chest. This focuses on draining toxins (specifically neurotoxins) from the central nervous system via the lymphatic system and into the blood, where they are then broken down in the liver. The technique also applies gentle pressure on the head, neck and back to support the flow of cerebrospinal fluid (CSF), removing blockages and enhancing the body's ability to restore homeo-stasis.

It is not aimed at curing disease but facilitates the body to 'self-correct'. A number of research studies are reviewing the Perrin Technique and it is also being investigated for supporting long-COVID patients.

The Lightning Process

The Lightning Process (LP) is a training programme that incorporates life coaching and NLP principles to help the body out of a persistent fight-or-flight response. It operates on the premise of the mind–body connection and how we can influence our physiology and health based upon improving mindset. It works by focusing on ways in which we might get 'stuck' in certain thought patterns and behaviours, helping us to shift our attention towards adapting and learning more positive and calmer ways of being, so as to settle the nervous system down once and for all.

The Lightning Process uses gentle movement, meditation-like tech-niques and mental exercises, which can change the way your nervous system works, switching on pathways that support health and switching off those that are unhelpful. You also gain skills on how to deal with negative situations involving your health and your life, which can be applied to helping you navigate CFS.

The LP is not endorsed by bodies such as the World ME Alliance; however, this does not mean that it cannot benefit CFS patients. I think the concern here is when patients might overexert themselves and worsen their symptoms as a result of changing their habits too rapidly, but, as long as habit change is done carefully and sensibly, it shouldn't pose any risk.

There are some other CFS-focused therapies that are thought to work in a similar manner to the LP, based upon the mind–body connection:

- The Gupta Program
- Mickel Therapy
- Reverse Therapy

Colonic Hydrotherapy

Colonic hydrotherapy, also known as colon cleansing or colonic irriga-tion, involves flushing the colon with fluids to remove waste. A tube is inserted into the rectum, that hydrates the bowel with warm, filtered water and flushes the waste away (it is said to cleanse, tone and exer-cise the colon). I like to view colonics as an internal bath that helps to provide a gentle internal massage and clear the colon of waste, gas, mucus and toxins. It also stimulates peristalsis, which encourages proper bowel function. The abdomen is massaged at stages throughout the colonic, too.

There aren't a huge number of studies to back colonic hydrotherapy just yet, but I have seen clients who have benefited from colonic treatments when it comes to fatigue, as well as the digestive troubles that accompany CFS. They can also be useful in detoxifying the body (particularly beneficial if toxicity is one of your chronic stressors) and hydrating the bowel, while loosening impacted waste that is stagnant. It is argued that colonics can flush away friendly bacteria in the gut, however any bacteria that is washed away can support microbial balance by eliminating disruptive microbes that take up residency, encouraging the beneficial communities to flourish. Plus, most of our gut bacteria are attached to the gut wall anyway, so they don't eliminate our entire ecosystem and it is not an intervention that is performed every day.

Enemas can also be performed alongside a colon cleanse. Water infused with herbal or nutritional compounds is held for a short period for 'retention' in the bowel to be absorbed and then the rest is evacu-ated. Enemas work on cleansing the lower colon, compared with colonics, which involve multiple infusions of water and target the whole colon. Examples include coffee, wheatgrass and probiotic enemas.

Reflexology

Reflexology is a type of massage involving the application of pressure to the feet and other body parts, such as the hands and ears. It is based on the theory that there are points in these areas (known as 'reflex points') that connect with certain organs and body systems and, when pressure is applied to them, it can improve energy flow within the body and provide health benefits. Although there isn't a huge body of evidence behind reflexology's ability to support CFS sufferers, per se, it can certainly assist the body's integral self-healing mechanisms through its ability to relax the nervous system and improve energy blocks within the body.

Acupuncture

Originally a component of ancient Chinese medicine, acupuncture involves the insertion of very fine needles into the skin at targeted areas on the body to improve the flow of energy. It has been shown to support the nervous system, particularly by stimulating the vagus nerve, and can promote the production of pain-relieving chemicals in the body, such as endorphins.

Hyperbaric oxygen therapy

Hyperbaric oxygen therapy is a treatment that takes place in a controlled and pressurised chamber to enhance the body's natural healing processes by providing it with more oxygen than normal. There have been some positive findings from studies regarding its ability to help reduce fatigue in CFS patients and long COVID, as well as supporting those with chronic pain (including fibromyalgia).

A variation of this is called ozone therapy, which works by administering ozone gas to the body to support oxygenation and restore health.

Other treatments

The following are also being investigated in relation to CFS:

- Apheresis (a method of filtering the blood to remove toxic components and infections)
- Chelation therapy (a way of removing heavy metals using a chelating agent)
- Chromotherapy (colour light therapy)
- Faecal transplants (the infusion of healthy donor faeces into the gut of a recipient to support the microbiome)

APPENDIX III

Further Support and Advice

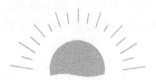

Tips for loved ones on how to support someone with CFS

If you have a friend or loved one with CFS, allow them to talk about their illness, and try to educate yourself about it, so that you can better grasp their situation and how things may have changed for them. Small gestures can help, such as sending a card when they are too unwell to see people, organising something nice that you are able to enjoy together, accompanying them to medical appointments, helping with cooking and shopping . . . And being understanding if they have to cancel arrangements because they are feeling unwell is important, too.

Tips for speaking to your boss or HR department to explain your situation

You may be surprised at how many of my clients have had supportive experiences at work, with employers agreeing to them going part-time, working from home or even taking a six-month sabbatical, allowing them the time they need to focus on some self-care and their health.

Seek out a supportive character who may be able to empathise with you. Explain how the illness is affecting you and your intention to do the best by your employer, given the circumstances. Ask questions about how your employer might be able to accommodate your health situation, so that you can still meet the requirements of your role.

Support from employers for chronically ill staff

If any of your staff members have CFS, try to find opportunities in the workplace to make things more manageable for them. This might involve things like designating a quiet area where they can work without too much stimulation and noise around them or ensuring that they have adequate rest breaks during the day. They might also benefit from work-from-home days when they are going through a crash in their CFS symptoms.

Applying for sickness benefits from the government

The government has schemes through which you can apply for sickness pay if you have a health condition that is affecting your ability to work (known as Employment and Support Allowance, or ESA), or, if your illness affects your ability to get around or perform everyday tasks (known as Personal Independence Payment, or PIP) – these can be very helpful if you are struggling financially (see Resources, p. 308).

Seeking the support of a healthcare practitioner

Seek the support of a healthcare professional (whether a nutritional therapist, naturopath, psychologist and/or CBT therapist or NLP practitioner) if you would like more help with implementing some of the practices in this book or to explore them in greater depth (see Resources, p. 308).

Recovery on a budget

There are undoubtedly financial implications when it comes to chronic illness and also from making the lifestyle changes that can help you to get well – and this is certainly something I can empathise with. So focus on what you can comfortably afford to take on from this book, and don't stress about what you cannot.

With lifestyle changes, prioritise what truly matters to you and what is relevant to where you are on your recovery journey. For example, you might want to regulate your sleep cycle as a starting point, and then look towards addressing any limiting beliefs that you have surrounding recovery being possible for you. You might, say, choose to concentrate on the mindfulness element of recovery and the pacing (see pp. 254 and

221), rather than fork out for expensive holistic therapies. In addition, there might be some underlying traumas or ACEs in your past that have not been dealt with, so you might look towards tapping, meditation and mindfulness practice to support recovery of the nervous system as you build the momentum in your healing.

When it comes to nutritional change, small steps really do count. For example, you might not be able to go 100 per cent organic, due to the expense, but you could, perhaps, set aside a budget towards some quality meat, eggs and fish every week. Simple shifts like cutting out ultra-processed and high-sugar foods can also achieve big wins with balancing hormones and supporting energy levels, so don't underestimate this. Also, you might not be able to eat three nutritionally balanced meals every single day, but aiming for one a day will give you a multitude of benefits over time that can then be built upon as you move forwards.

Time is also a key resource when it comes to recovery – we must never underestimate its power for healing and recovery; and, best of all, it's free. Patience with the time that recovery takes is something you must become well acquainted with, as it helps you to reclaim your health.

Focus on your identity outside of illness
It is so important to value yourself based on all your positive attributes and not see yourself solely through the lens of your illness. I often see chronically unwell patients who get lost behind labels like CFS/ME/Lyme/MCS/MCAS, when this is really just an alphabet soup at the end of the day. Don't let illness become your sole identity. It might be a part of you (for the time being), but it does not define you.

Navigating medical appointments
Keep a diary of your symptoms to take to your GP or other medical appointments. If you find that you need more time communicating your problems or that the drain on your energy may be too high, why not book a double appointment and take a friend or relative with you for support. They can help you to communicate your main points to the GP and note down or remember the main points of information.

APPENDIX IV

Recovery Checklist

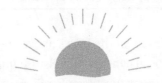

I have compiled a checklist for the different avenues explored in this book that you can tick off if and as you are completing them to ensure that you are covering some of the key bases to support recovery.

Don't feel overwhelmed. Instead, see this checklist as providing some structure to your recovery process and keeping you on track. You may wish to try some of them at different stages, and others by working on them simultaneously.

Recovery checklist	✔
Read this book.	
Consulted a doctor about symptoms.	
Worked with a nutritionist, naturopath or functional-medicine practitioner who has experience working with CFS.	
Explored functional testing with a practitioner.	
Explored dietary changes and supplements, if necessary.	
Worked on improving gut health.	
Removed toxic products from my home and switched to natural ones.	
Reduced exposure to environmental toxins, such as moulds, heavy metals, pesticides.	
Established a solid sleep routine.	
Incorporated pacing and, when the time was right, gently graded my level of physical activity.	

Practised NLP and CBT techniques.	
Reduced macro- and micro-stressors to balance my nervous system.	
Explored complementary therapies (say, the Perrin Technique).	
Practised regular journaling to work through emotions and mindset.	
Explored my beliefs about recovery.	
Took regular Epsom-salt baths.	
Worked on supporting my detoxification systems.	

Note: if you have ticked all the boxes above and are still struggling to see progress, do not be alarmed – this list is simply to ensure that you have covered most of the major lifestyle pillars of recovery.

GLOSSARY

Acupuncture: an alternative therapy that involves inserting fine needles into the skin at specific points

Adrenal glands: two glands that sit above the kidneys and secrete cortisol and adrenaline

Adrenal insufficiency: where the adrenals have been under stress due to a long-term fight-or-flight response and fail to produce adequate stress hormones (such as cortisol) as a result

Allergy: a damaging immune response to a particular substance (known as an allergen); this could be a food, chemical, dust, pollen or animal fur, for example

Anaemia: a deficiency (or dysfunction) of red blood cells, reducing the delivery of oxygen to the body's tissues (it is a common driver of fatigue)

Antioxidants: molecules found in various foods (particularly vegetables) and produced in the body; they help to protect cells against damage from oxidation (the loss of electrons by a molecule in a reaction)

Aromatherapy: the use of aromatic plant extracts and essential oils for therapeutic and medicinal purposes

Autoimmune disease: where the immune system mistakes bodily tissue for an antigen (a foreign substance that induces an immune response) and attacks itself as a result

Autoimmune protocol (AIP): a diet that removes foods that might aggravate autoimmune-disease symptoms and chronic illness

Autonomic nervous system (ANS): the involuntary branch of the peripheral nervous system, which controls heart rate, breathing, digestion and body temperature; it is divided into the enteric, parasympathetic and sympathetic nervous systems

Boom-and-bust cycle: the ups and downs of activity during CFS, in which patients tend to expend too much energy when their symptoms are at bay (boom), resulting in post-exertional malaise (bust)

Candida albicans: an opportunistic pathogenic yeast that resides within the gut microbiome (as well as the mouth and vagina); Candida can overgrow and lead to chronic health problems (it has been associated with CFS)

Chronic fatigue syndrome (CFS): a chronic illness that affects multiple body systems, including the nervous, endocrine, immune and digestive systems and mitochondria

Circadian rhythm: the natural internal process (or twenty-four-hour cycle) that regulates our sleep and wakefulness

Cognitive behavioural therapy (CBT): a talking therapy that helps to support changes to the way people think and behave; it is based upon the concept that your thoughts, feelings, physical sensations and actions are all connected

Commensalism: an association between two microorganisms where one benefits and the other derives neither benefit or harm

Co-morbidity: a disease or medical condition that is present alongside another (or multiple others)

Cortisol: the body's main stress hormone, produced by the adrenal glands

Cytokines: small proteins released by cells (including immune cells) to coordinate the body's response to infection, triggering inflammation

Detoxification: the process of removing toxic substances from the body

Disorder: an impairment in bodily structure or function (either physical or mental) – for example, an arrhythmia (irregular heartbeat) is a type of heart disorder

Dysautonomia: a disorder where the autonomic nervous system (ANS) does not work as it should

Dysbiosis: an imbalance between the beneficial and potentially harmful microorganisms present within a person's microbiome, especially that of the gut, which can have a negative impact on overall health

Dysregulation: the term used to describe how physiological and meta-bolic processes can become impaired in CFS, which helps us to better understand the illness

Enteric nervous system (ENS): the network of nerves within the digest-ive system that help to control various functions

Enzyme: a type of protein that assists chemical reactions in the body

Fibre: a type of carbohydrate that is resistant to the action of digestive enzymes, so the human body cannot digest it; however, fibre acts as a food source for beneficial types of bacteria in the gut microbiome, which can benefit human health

FODMAP: fermentable oligo-, di-, monosaccharides and polyols – types of carbohydrates (sugars) that can be fermented by the bacteria in the human gut, often giving rise to digestive symptoms (particularly IBS)

Food allergy: an (often severe) immune response (that involves IgE antibodies) towards a food protein

Food intolerance: a reaction to a food that is often related to a problem with mechanically breaking food down in the digestive system or an enzyme deficiency, or a problem where the gut microbes ferment a food component

Food sensitivity: an immune response to a food protein involving IGG antibodies (it can be silent in some cases); food sensitivity can lead to a leaky gut

Free radical: an unstable molecule with an unpaired electron

Functional medicine: a physiology- and systems-based approach that focuses on identifying and addressing the root causes of chronic disease

Functional testing: a method of testing the body for how well it is functioning

Gluten: a type of protein found in grains such as wheat, barley, rye and spelt

Glymphatic system: a network of lymphatic vessels that clear waste from the central nervous system, mostly when we sleep

Histamine intolerance: a build-up of histamine in the body and an inability to eliminate it

Homeostasis: a tendency to achieve equilibrium (a state of balance) within the body's physiology

HPA axis: hypothalamic–pituitary–adrenal axis

HPT axis: hypothalamic–pituitary–thyroid axis

Hypothalamus: the body's hormone command centre within the brain; it coordinates with the pituitary gland

Inflammation: a process involved in fighting off injury or infection; the problem is when it becomes chronic

Leaky gut: when the cells that line the gut wall become permeable (also known as 'intestinal permeability')

Lightning Process: a training system that provides tools (based on life coaching and NLP) to support the health of the nervous system

Long COVID: a long-term illness resulting from a SARS-CoV-2 infection, which features chronic fatigue and runs parallel with CFS

Macro-stressors: significant life stressors that we have less influence over

Microbiome: the entire population of microorganisms (including their genes) within a certain area on or in the body

Microbiota: the microbes that exist within a particular environment (for example, the gut microbiota)

Micro-stressors: small common stress triggers that often occur daily, and over which we have more influence

Mindfulness: the ability to become fully present and aware of what we are doing within a given moment, without forming judgement or opinions

Mitochondria: organelles within cells that produce a chemical called ATP (adenosine triphosphate) – the body's energy currency compound

Mutualism: a relationship between two microorganisms where each species derives benefits from the other

Myalgic encephalomyelitis (ME): another name for CFS, given after an outbreak at the Royal Free Hospital in London in 1955

Mycobiome: the fungal communities in or on a particular area of the body (notably in the gut)

Naturopathy: a system of alternative medicine based on the theory that diseases can successfully be supported or prevented through interventions such as diet, lifestyle, movement, herbs and supplements; the philosophy of naturopathy runs parallel to functional medicine

Nervous system: the body's command centre, which coordinates much of what we think and feel, as well as actions that the body carries out

Neuroendocrine system: where the nervous and endocrine systems meet to produce and secrete hormones

Neuro-linguistic programming (NLP): a way of examining and influencing how our thoughts and language patterns shape our behaviour, based upon the belief that our thoughts can be reprogrammed for more positive behavioural and health outcomes

Neurotransmitter: a chemical messenger in the body

Nocebo: the opposite of a placebo response – where thinking that something will harm you produces a negative effect

Organic acids test: a urine test that examines metabolic by-products

Oxidative stress: an imbalance between antioxidants and free radicals in the body

Pacing: an approach that involves striking a balance between levels of activity and rest

Parasites: organisms that make up the microbiome which can become opportunistic and cause chronic health problems

Parasympathetic nervous system (PNS): a branch of the autonomic nervous system (ANS) that governs the relaxation response (also known as the 'rest-and-digest' mode)

Pathophysiology: the physiological processes in the body affected within a particular disease

Post-exertional malaise (PEM): a form of fatigue in CFS that occurs upon exertion (particularly after exercise or physical activity, but also from mental and emotional activity beyond one's threshold); PEM is a key symptom for the majority of CFS sufferers

Prebiotics: fermentable, indigestible compounds in food that act as a food source for our friendly bacteria to consume and gain nourishment

Presuppositions: an NLP tool that offers a more helpful way of viewing the world around us

Probiotics: live microorganisms that, when consumed in adequate quantities, confer certain health benefits

Psychoneuroendocrinoimmunology: the interaction between our thoughts and the functioning of our nervous, endocrine and immune systems

Rapid eye movement sleep (REM): a stage of sleep occurring after deep sleep, which is associated with dreaming and memory consolidation

Reflexology: an alternative massage therapy using reflex points on the feet, hands and head that are said to be linked to the rest of the body

Small intestinal bacterial overgrowth (SIBO): a form of dysbiosis where bacteria are present in the small intestine

Stress: a state of strain or tension resulting from adverse or demanding circumstances (this can be physical or psychological)

Submodalities: the finer distinctions we make within a representational system – for example, a picture could be black and white or colour, or it could also be bright or dim; sounds can be loud or soft, or coming from a particular direction

Sympathetic nervous system (SNS): the part of the autonomic nervous system (ANS) that produces the fight-or-flight response

Syndrome: a group of symptoms that consistently occur together

Toxin: any substance that is harmful or poisonous to the body

Trauma: a stressful experience that activates a robust emotional response

Virome: a term used to describe the assemblage of viruses that are found in and on the human body

RESOURCES

Where to find me
ARDERE: www.ardere.com
Shop: www.ardere.com/product-category/collection/shop
Practitioner website: www.laurenwindas.com

Functional lab testing
(**Note:** functional testing can be arranged via a nutritional-therapy practitioner.)
Genova Diagnostics: www.gdx.net/uk
ArminLabs: www.arminlabs.com/en
   (UK ArminLabs contact: www.aonm.org)
Lifecode GX: www.lifecodegx.com
Regenerus Labs: www.regeneruslabs.com

CFS charities
The ME Association: www.meassociation.org.uk
Action for M.E.: www.actionforme.org.uk

CFS research trials
Decode ME Study: www.decodeme.org.uk

Healthy meal box delivery
Mindful Chef: www.mindfulchef.com
Detox Kitchen: www.detoxkitchen.co.uk

Organic food suppliers
Riverford: www.riverford.co.uk
Abel & Cole: www.abelandcole.co.uk

Mindfulness
www.positivepsychology.com/mindfulness-exercises-techniques-activities
www.healthline.com/health/how-to-use-mala-beads#takeaway

Meditation
Insight Timer: www.insighttimer.com/en-gb

Breathwork
Breathwork exercises: www.verywellmind.com/abdominal-
breathing-2584115
Flourish – Guided Breathwork app: www.thebreathguy.com/online.html
Wim Hof Method breathwork app: www.wimhofmethod.com/
wim-hof-method-mobile-app

Cognitive behavioural therapy (CBT) tools and techniques
www.positivepsychology.com/cbt-cognitive-behavioral-therapy-
techniques-worksheets

Emotional freedom technique (EFT or tapping)
www.thetappingsolution.com/tapping-101 and download their 'Tapping
Solution' app

Healthcare Practitioners
Nutritional therapy: www.practitioner-search.bant.org.uk
Naturopathy practitioners: www.gncouncil.co.uk
NLP practitioners: www.anlp.org/member-search
Psychologists: British psychological society: www.bps.org.uk/find-
psychologist

Government support
Claiming sickness benefit: www.gov.uk/browse/benefits/disability

Miscellaneous
British Society for Mercury Free Dentistry: www.mercuryfreedentistry.
org.uk/london-south
Environmental Working Group (EWG) Skin Deep Cosmetics Database:
www.ewg.org/skindeep
Discover your chronotype: www.cet-surveys.com/index.
php?sid=61524&newtest=Y

The sunflower lanyard: those with invisible disabilities can apply for a sunflower lanyard from www.hiddendisabilitiesstore.com – a UK-based company that aims to spread awareness and understanding of invisible illness, the idea being that wearing the sunflower lanyard will help others to recognise your condition when you are travelling.

REFERENCES

Part 2

1. Hvidberg, M.F., Brinth, L.S., Oelsen, A.V., Petersen, K.D. and Ehlers, L. (2015). 'The health-related quality of life for patients with myalgic encephalomyelitis / chronic fatigue syndrome (ME/CFS)', *PLoS One*, 10 (7). doi: 10.1371/journal.pone.0132421

2. Stevelink, S.A.M., Fear, N.T., Hotopf, M. and Chalder, T. (2019). 'Factors associated with work status in chronic fatigue syndrome', *Occupational Medicine*, 69 (6). doi: 10.1093/occmed/kqz108.

3. NICE (2021). 'Myalgic encephalomyelitis (or encephalopathy)/ chronic fatigue syndrome: diagnosis and management'. Available at: https://www.nice.org.uk/guidance/ng206/resources/ myalgic-encephalomyelitis-or-encephalopathychronic-fatigue-syn-drome-diagnosis-and-management-pdf-66143718094021

4. Griffith, J.P. and Zarrouf, F.A. (2008). 'A Systematic Review of Chronic Fatigue Syndrome: Don't Assume It's Depression', *Primary Care Companion to the Journal of Clinical Psychiatry*, 10 (2), pp. 120–128. doi: 10.4088/pcc.v10n0206

5. Devasahayam, A., Lawn, T. and White, P.D. (2012). 'Alternative diagnoses to chronic fatigue syndrome in referrals to a specialist service: service evaluation survey', *Journal of the Royal Society of Medicine*, 3 (1). doi: 10.1258/shorts.2011.011127

6. It should be noted that GET and CBT are not without their criticisms; for example, GET no longer forms part of the UK's healthcare guidelines.

7. Forward-ME. (2019). 'Evaluation of a survey exploring the experiences of adults and children with ME/CFS who have participated in CBT and GET interventional programmes', The ME Association Available at: https://meassociation.org.uk/wp-content/uploads NICE-Patient-Survey-Outcomes-CBT-and-GET-Executive-Summary-from-Forward-ME-03.04.19.pdf

8. Buchwald, D., Herrell, R., Ashton, S., Belcourt, M., Schmaling,

K., Sullivan, P., Neale, M. and Goldberg, J. (2001). 'A twin study of chronic fatigue', *Psychosomatic Medicine*, 63, pp. 936–943. doi: 10.1097/00006842-200111000-00012

9. Lande, A., Fluge, Ø., Strand, E.B., Flåm, S.T., Sosa, D.D., Mella, O., Egeland, T., Saugstad, O.D., Lie, B.A. and Viken, M.K. (2020). 'Human Leukocyte Antigen alleles associated with Myalgic Encephalomyelitis/Chronic Fatigue Syndrome (ME/CFS)', *Scientific Reports*, 10 (5267). doi: 10.1038/s41598-020-62157-x

10. Decode ME. (2023). *Decode ME: the ME/CFS study*. Available at: https://www.decodeme.org.uk/decodeme-dna-study-awarded-3m-funding

11. Salit, E. (1997). 'Precipitating factors for the chronic fatigue syndrome', *Journal of Psychiatric Research*, 31 (1), pp. 59–65. doi: 10.1016/s0022-3956(96)00050-7

12. Appel, S., Chapman, J. and Shoenfeld, Y. (2007). 'Infection and vaccination in chronic fatigue syndrome: myth or reality?', *Autoimmunity*, 40 (1), pp. 48–53. doi: 10.1080/08916930701197273

13. Vermeulen, R.C.W. and Scholte, H.R. (2003). 'Rupture of silicone gel breast implants and symptoms of pain and fatigue', *The Journal of Rheumatology*, 30 (10), pp. 2263–2267, PubMed [Online]. Available at: https://pubmed.ncbi.nlm.nih.gov/14528527

14. Racciatti, D., Vecchiet, J., Ceccomancini, A., Ricci, F. and Pizzigallo, E. 'Chronic fatigue syndrome following a toxic exposure', *Science of the Total Environment*, 270 (1–3), pp. 27–31. doi: 10.1016/s0048-9697(00)00777-4

15. Van Cauwenbergh, D., Nijs, J., Kos, D., Van Weijnen, L., Struyf, F. and Meeus, M. (2014). 'Malfunctioning of the autonomic nervous system in patients with chronic fatigue syndrome: a systematic literature review', *European Journal of Clinical Investigation*, 44 (5), pp. 516–526. doi: 10.1111/eci.12256

16. Demitrack, M.A., Dale, J.K., Straus, S.E., Laue, L., Listwak, S.J., Kruesi, M.J.P., Chrousos, G.P. and Gold, P.W. (1991). 'Evidence for Impaired Activation of the Hypothalamic-Pituitary-Adrenal Axis in Patients with Chronic Fatigue Syndrome', *The Journal of Clinical Endocrinology & Metabolism*, 73 (6), pp. 1224–1234. doi: 10.1210/jcem-73-6-1224

17. Papadopoulos, A.S. and Cleare, A.J. (2012). 'Hypothalamic-pituitary-adrenal axis dysfunction in chronic fatigue syndrome', *Nature Reviews Endocrinology*, 8 (1), pp.22–32. doi: 10.1038/nrendo.2011.153

18. Ruiz-Núñez, B., Tarasse, R., Vogelaar, E.F., Dijck-Brouwer, D.A.J. and Muskiet, F.A.J. (2018). 'Higher prevalence of "low T3 syndrome" in patients with chronic fatigue syndrome: a case-control study', *Frontiers in Endocrinology*, 9 (97). doi: 10.3389/fendo.2018.00097

19. Jacobs, J.J.L. (2021). 'Persistent SARS-2 infections contribute to long COVID-19', *Medical Hypotheses*, 149. doi: 10.1016%2Fj.mehy.2021.110538

20. Montoya, J.G., Holmes, T.H., Anderson, J.N. and Davis, M.M. (2017). 'Cytokine signature associated with disease severity in chronic fatigue syndrome patients', *Proceedings of the National Academy of Sciences*, 114 (34). doi: 10.1073/pnas.1710519114

21. Bates, D.W., Buchwald, D., Lee, J., Kith, P., Doolittle, T., Rutherford, C., Churchill, W.H., Schur, P.H., Wener, M., Wybenga, D., Winkelman, J. and Komaroff, A.L. (1995). 'Clinical laboratory test findings in patients with chronic fatigue syndrome', *Archives of Internal Medicine*, 155 (1), pp. 97–103. doi: 10.1001/archinte.1995.00430010105014

22. Schoeman E.M., Van Der Westhuizen, F.H., Erasmus, E., Van Dyk, E., Knowles, C.V.Y., Al-Ali, S., Ng, W.F., Taylor, R.W., Newton, J.L. and Elson, J.L. (2017). 'Clinically proven mtDNA mutations are not common in those with chronic fatigue syndrome', *BMC Medical Genetics*, 18 (29). doi: 10.1186/s12881-017-0387-6

23. Castro-Marrero, J., Cordero, M.D., Sáez-Francas, N., Jimenez-Gutierrez, C., Aguilar-Montilla, F.J., Aliste, L. and Alegre-Martin, J. (2013). 'Could Mitochondrial Dysfunction Be a Differentiating Marker Between Chronic Fatigue Syndrome and Fibromyalgia?', *Antioxidants and Redox Signalling*, 19 (15). doi: 10.1089/ars.2013.5346

24. Thomas, C., Brown, A., Strassheim, V., Elson, J.L., Newton, J. and Manning, P. (2018). 'Cellular bioenergetics is impaired in patients with chronic fatigue syndrome', *PLoS ONE*, 13 (2). doi: 10.1371/journal.pone.0192817.

25. Aaron, L.A., Burke, M.M. and Buchwald, D. (2000). 'Overlapping conditions among patients with chronic fatigue syndrome, fibromyalgia, and temporomandibular disorder', *The Archives of Internal Medicine*, 160 (2), pp. 221–227. doi: 10.1001/archinte.160.2.221

26. Allen-Vercoe, E. and Petrof, E.O. (2014). 'The microbiome: what it means for medicine', *British Journal of General Practice*, 64 (620), pp. 188–119. doi: 10.3399/bjgp14X677374

27. Beaumont, A., Burton, A.R., Lemon, J., Bennett, B.K., Lloyd, A. and Vollmer-Conna, U. (2012). 'Reduced Cardiac Vagal Modulation Impacts on Cognitive Performance in Chronic Fatigue Syndrome', *PLoS ONE*, 7 (11). doi: 10.1371/journal.pone.0049518

28. Giloteaux, L., Goodrich, J.K., Walters, W.A., Levine, S.M., Ley, R.E. and Hanson, M.R. (2016). 'Reduced diversity and altered composition of the gut microbiome in individuals with myalgic encephalomyelitis/chronic fatigue syndrome', *Microbiome*, 4, pp. 953–959. doi: 10.1186/s40168-016-0171-4

29. Frémont, M., Coomans, D., Massart, S. and De Meirleir, K. (2013). 'High-throughput 16S rRNA gene sequencing reveals alterations of intestinal microbiota in myalgic encephalomyelitis/chronic fatigue syndrome patients', *Anaerobe*, 22, pp. 50–56. doi: 10.1016/j.anaerobe.2013.06.002

30. Nagy-Szakal, D., Williams, B.L., Mishra, N., Che, X., Lee, B., Bateman, L., Klimas, N.G., Komaroff, A.L., Levine, S., Montoya, J.G., Peterson, D.L., Ramanan, D., Jain, K., Eddy, ML., Hornig, M. and Lipkin, W.I. (2017). 'Fecal metagenomic profiles in subgroups of patients with myalgic encephalomyelitis/ chronic fatigue syndrome', *Microbiome*, 5 (44). doi: 10.1186/s40168-017-0261-y

31. Heim, C., Nater, U.M., Maloney, E., Boneva, R., Jones, J.F. and Reeves, W.C. (2009). 'Childhood Trauma and Risk for Chronic fatigue Syndrome: Association with Neuroendocrine Dysfunction', *Archives of General Psychiatry*, 66 (1), pp. 72–80. doi: 10.1001/archgenpsychiatry.2008.508

32. De Lemos, E.T., Oliveira, J., Pinheiro, J.P. and Reis, F. (2012). 'Regular Physical Exercise as a Strategy to Improve Antioxidant and Anti-Inflammatory Status: Benefits in Type 2 Diabetes Mellitus', *Oxidative Medicine and Cellular Longevity*. doi: 10.1155/2012/741545

33. Heap, L.C., Peters, T.J. and Wessely, S. (1999). 'Vitamin B status in patients with chronic fatigue syndrome', *Journal of the Royal Society of Medicine*, 92 (4), pp. 183–185. doi: 10.1177/014107689909200405

34. Jacobson, W., Saich, T., Borysiewicz, L.K., Behan, W.M.H., Behan, P.O. and Wreghitt, T.G., (1993). 'Serum folate and chronic fatigue syndrome', *Neurology*, 43 (12), pp. 2645–2647. doi: 10.1212/WNL.43.12.2645

35. Cox, I.M., Campbell, M.J. and Dowson, D. (1991). 'Red blood cell magnesium and chronic fatigue syndrome', *Lancet*, 337 (8744), pp. 757–7690. doi: 10.1016/0140-6736(91)91371-z

36. Plioplys, A.V. and Plioplys, S. (1995). 'Serum Levels of Carnitine in

Chronic Fatigue Syndrome: Clinical Correlates', *Neuropsychobiology*, 32, pp. 132–138. doi: 10.1159/000119226

37. Maes, M., Mihaylova, I., Kubera, M., Uytterhoeven, M., Vrydags, N. and Bosmans, E. (2009). 'Coenzyme Q10 deficiency in myalgic encephalomyelitis/chronic fatigue syndrome (ME/CFS) is related to fatigue, autonomic and neurocognitive symptoms and is another risk factor explaining the early mortality in ME/CFS due to cardiovascular disorder', 30 (4), pp. 470–476, PubMed [Online]. Available at: https://pubmed.ncbi.nlm.nih.gov/20010505

38. Kurup, R.K. and Kurup, P.A. (2003). 'Hypothalamic digoxin, cerebral chemical dominance and myalgic encephalomyelitis', 113 (5), pp. 683–701. doi: 10.1080/00207450390200026

39. Castro-Marrero, J., Zaragozá, M.C., Domingo, J.C., Martinez-Martinez, A., Alegre, J. and Von Schacky, C. (2018). 'Low omega-3 index and polyunsaturated fatty acid status in patients with chronic fatigue syndrome/myalgic encephalomyelitis', *Prostaglandins, Leukotrienes & Essential Fatty Acids*, 139, pp. 20–24. doi: 10.1016/j.plefa.2018.11.006

Part Three

1. Fasano, A., Sapone, A., Zevallos, V. and Schuppan, D. (2015). 'Nonceliac Gluten Sensitivity', *Gastroenterology*, 148 (6), pp. 1195–1204. doi: 10.1053/j.gastro.2014.12.049

2. Krysiak, R., Szkróbka, W. and Okopień, B. (2019). 'The Effect of Gluten-Free Diet on Thyroid Autoimmunity in Drug-Naïve Women with Hashimoto's Thyroiditis: A Pilot Study', *Experimental and Clinical Endocrinology and Diabetes*, 127 (7). pp. 417–422. doi: 10.1055/a-0653-7108

3. Lerner, A., Shoenfeld, Y. and Matthias, T. (2017). 'Adverse effects of gluten ingestion and advantages of gluten withdrawal in nonceliac autoimmune disease', *Nutrition Reviews*, 75 (12), pp. 1046–1058. doi: 10.1093/nutrit/nux054

4. Hollon, J., Puppa, E.L., Greenwald, B., Goldberg, E., Guerrerio, A. and Fasano, A. (2015). 'Effect of Gliadin on Permeability of Intestinal Biopsy Explants from Celiac Disease Patients and Patients with Non-Celiac Gluten Sensitivity', *Nutrients*, 7 (3), pp. 1565–1576. doi: 10.3390/nu7031565

5. Mahboubi, M. (2020). 'Sambucus Nigra (Black Elder) as Alternative Treatment for Cold and Flu', *Advances in Traditional Medicine*, 21, pp. 405–414. doi: 10.1007/s13596-020-00469-z

6. Feng, J., Leone, J., Schweig, S. and Zhang, Y. (2020). 'Evaluation of

Natural and Botanical Medicines for Activity Against Growing and Non-growing Forms of B. burgdorferi', *Frontiers in Medicine*, 7 . doi: 10.3389/fmed.2020.00006

7. Ibid.

8. Tarozzi, A., Angeloni, C., Malaguti, M., Morroni, F., Hrelia, S. and Hrelia, P. (2013). 'Sulforaphane as a Potential Protective Phytochemical against Neurodegenerative Diseases', *Oxidative Medicine and Cellular Longevity*. doi: 10.1155/2013/415078

9. Calder, P.C. (2010). 'Omega 3 fatty acids and inflammatory processes', Nutrients, 2 (3), pp. 355–374. doi: 10.3390/nu2030355

10. Promdam, N. and Panichayupakaranant, P. (2022). '[6]-Gingerol: A narrative review of its beneficial effect on human health', *Food Chemistry Advances*, 1. doi: 10.1016/j.focha.2022.100043

11. Hewlings, S.J. and Kalman, D.S. (2017). 'Curcumin: a review of its effects on human health', *Foods*, 6 (10). doi: 10.3390/foods6100092

12. Santinelli, L., Laghi, L., Innocenti, G.P., Pinacchio, C., Vassalini, P., Celani, L., Lazzaro, A., Borrazzo, C., Marazzato, M., Tarsitani, L., Koukopoulos, A.E., Mastroianni, C.M., d'Ettorre, G. and Ceccarelli, G. (2022). 'Oral bacteriotherapy reduces the occurrence of chronic fatigue in COVID-19 patients', *Frontiers in Nutrition*, 8. doi: 10.3389/fnut.2021.756177

13. Rao, R. and Samak, G. (2015). 'Role of glutamine in protection of intestinal epithelial tight junctions', *Journal of Epithelial Biology & Pharmacology*, 5. doi: 10.2174/1875044301205010047

14. Cigna (2019). 'Chronic stress; are we reaching health system burnout'. Available at: https://www.cignaglobal.com/static/docs/pdf/cigna-asia-care-report-18-nov.pdf

15. ME Research UK. (2016). *ME/CFS research funding*. Available at: https://www.meresearch.org.uk/wp-content/uploads/2016/09/mecfs-research-funding-report-2016-final.pdf

ACKNOWLEDGEMENTS

There isn't a shadow of a doubt in my mind who I have to thank for getting me to where I am today.

To Mum, Dad and my sister, Nicole – for all your love and support. For being there for me through the years as times got tough. When I didn't know how I would go on at the crux of my illness, words cannot express how much it meant to have you there, fully understanding and there to ride the waves with me through each and every step.

Dad, I couldn't have asked for a parent more supportive than you. You gave me a comfort blanket to fall back on and solace in knowing that I would get well, no matter what it took. You coached me mentally, made me laugh at times when I needed it the most and were always on the other end of a phone, cheering me on and saying how proud you were of me. You helped Nicole and me to build ARDERE into what it is today, with your passion, creative ingenuity and unwavering belief in your two daughters. Having had a close relationship like ours is something that I will cherish in my heart for ever. You are and will always be my hero. Not a day goes by when I don't miss you, your zest for life and enthusiastic spirit. This book is dedicated to you, the best dad I could have ever asked for. I love you.

Mum, quite simply, you are the best. Your energy and ability to empathise are irreplaceable. I couldn't meet a more caring person even if I tried. For those nights you stayed up worried sick about your youngest daughter, researching answers and fighting the battles for me with medical naysayers, at times when I couldn't muster up the energy to do the same. Thank you. Your wisdom and support have been a key driving force throughout this whole journey. You've held my hand, wiped my tears, cooked delicious healthy meals and found me the right support wherever necessary. Your calming energy inspires me. I'm so grateful that you get to be my mum.

Nicole, my sister and other half. We've walked through so much of life together, arm in arm. You've been there during the toughest of times when my health was at its worst and I couldn't see a way out. Being able to build a business with you has been the biggest blessing, as I've seen you grow into the most amazing businesswoman who inspires me on a daily basis. A sounding board to my anxieties, you've always picked me up when I've been down. You've pushed and encouraged me every day to get this book finished, and it would not be possible without you helping to make it happen. To my biggest cheerleader and best friend in the world. Thank you for everything.

Thank you also to my incredibly strong clients for teaching me so much through their own health journeys and inspiring me in the process.

A big thank you to the most supportive publishers. To Liv Nightingall, Liz Gough and Emma Knight at Yellow Kite, my brilliant editor Anne Newman and my literary agent Clare Hulton for their ongoing support, patience and guidance along the journey of writing this book; I can't thank you enough.

And finally, to my love, Chris, for never seeing me as anything other than myself. For listening, understanding and always nudging me towards achieving my goals. For being there during the tough times and having an incredible ability to make me laugh in almost any given situation – you are my world.

RECIPE INDEX

INDEX

terrain theory 90
testing: food-reactivity 130
  functional 112–23
  GP tests 114–15
thought journals 276–8
thought patterns 261–3, 267
thyroid gland 53–4, 55–6, 79, 129
  goitrogen 151, 161
  and the gut 72, 77
  hypo- and hyperthyroidism 55, 56, 117
  iodine and 166–7
  and soya intake 151
  testing thyroid function 113
  thyroid dysfunction 115, 117
thyroid hormones 53–4, 55, 167, 168
thyroid-stimulating hormone (TSH) 54, 55
thyroxine (T4) 54, 55, 72
time-restricted eating 158–60
timeline, health 91–2
tiredness, types of 233
toilet habits 241
toluene 243
tomatoes: Greek salad with soft-boiled eggs 198
  ratatouille with tender chicken thighs 202–3
  spicy scrambled eggs with heirloom tomato salad, smoked salmon and kimchi 183–4
tortillas, Mexican-spiced turkey 206–7
toxins 78–92, 158
  detoxification 118, 240–6
  reducing your toxic load 244–6
  toxicity testing 116, 122
trans fats 145, 150–1
trauma 79, 81–8, 280–1
traybake, salmon and vegetable 200–1
triclosan 243
triggers, precipitating 37, 38–9, 44
triiodothyronine (T3) 54, 55, 72

turkey: Mexican-spiced turkey tortillas 206–7
turmeric 166
  coconut and flax turmeric 'porridge' with stewed apple 181

ultra-processed foods 145, 148–9, 300
unwinding 251

vagus nerve 71–2, 297
vegeree 203–4
vegetables 146, 147, 170
  beef and root vegetable stew 210
  cruciferous vegetables 160–1
  green leafy vegetables 160
  salmon and vegetable traybake 200–1
ventilation 244
Vietnamese prawn summer rolls 196–7
viruses 58, 75, 77, 90
vitamins 118, 121, 179
  B vitamins 88, 89, 119, 121, 141, 149, 150, 161–2
  vitamin C 119, 168
  vitamin D 119, 256
  vitamin testing 119–20

water 172–3, 244
well-formed outcomes (WFOs) 268–9
wheat 126, 138
  wheat allergy (WA) 139
wi-fi 246
wired-and-tired stage 103–4, 215, 219–20, 221, 236
wormwood 152

yeast 126
yoghurt, passion fruit and pomegranate quick-serve 187

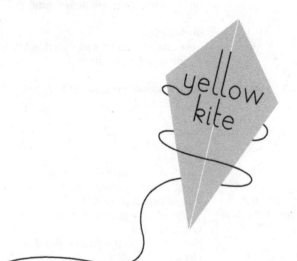

books to help you live a good life

Join the conversation and tell
us how you live a #goodlife

🐦 @yellowkitebooks
f YellowKiteBooks
𝓟 Yellow Kite Books
📷 YellowKiteBooks